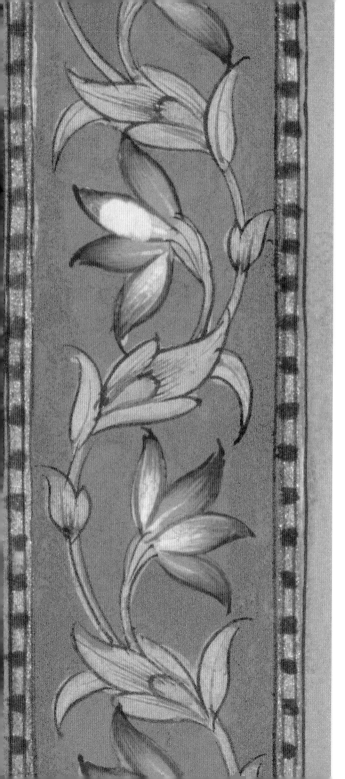

Simply
Ayurveda

Discover your Type to Transform
your Life

Bharti Vyas

with Jane Warren

Thorsons

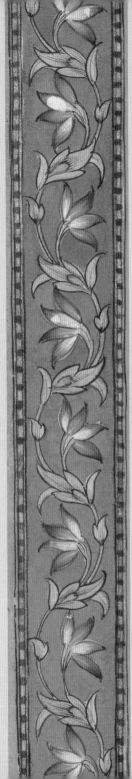

Note to the reader

The remedies and techniques described in *Simply Ayurveda* are meant to supplement, not be a substitute for, professional medical care or treatment. Although the teachings of Ayurveda are an excellent lifestyle adjunct, they should not be used to treat a serious ailment without prior consultation with a doctor. If you think someone in your family may be seriously ill please contact your GP or local hospital.

Thorsons
An Imprint of HarperCollins*Publishers*
77–85 Fulham Palace Road,
Hammersmith, London W6 8JB

The Thorsons website address is: www.thorsons.com

Published by Thorsons 2000

10 9 8 7 6 5 4 3 2 1

© Bharti Vyas 2000

Bharti Vyas, Jane Warren and Jeannette Ewin assert the moral right to
be identified as the authors of this work

Design: Jacqui Caulton
Editor: Lizzy Gray
Photography: Dave King
Photographs page 91: Robin Matthews
Illustrations pages 9, 119, 131 and decorative motifs courtesy of Victoria & Albert Museum

A catalogue record for this book
is available from the British Library

ISBN 0 7225 4028 0

Printed in Hong Kong by
Midas Printing (UK) Ltd.

Contents

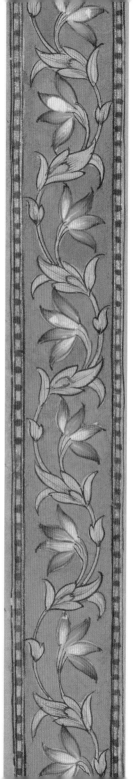

Part One: Ayurveda - The Science
    of Life

Introduction 4
Ayurvedic Dosha Questionnaire
    17
Vata – Air 27
Pitta – Fire 33
Kapha– Earth 39

Part Two: Ayurvedic Healing - Mind,
    Body and Soul

Beauty 46
Ayurveda and Women 60
Supplements 68
A–Z of Common Ailments 74
Yoga, Meditation & Breathing 84
Body Purification 104
Sexuality 124

Part Three: Balancing your Life
    through Food and Water

Ayurveda and Nutrition 136
Recipes 143
Foods to Balance Air 170
Foods to Balance Fire 173
Foods to Balance Earth 176

Resources 179
Further Reading 183
Index 185

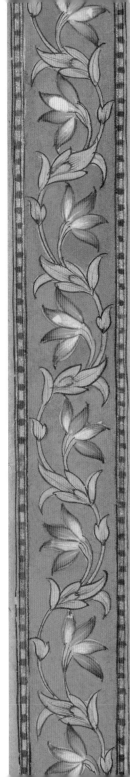

Dedication

I would like to dedicate this book to all my well-wishers, clients, readers and worldwide visitors to my website without whose support, encouragement and belief in my philosophies I could not have produced this book.

A special thanks goes firstly to my talented co-author Jane Warren and her supportive husband Willem Mulder. Also to Dr Jeannette Ewin the wonderful nutritionist and cookery writer for her contribution.

Acknowledgements

To my late and loving parents Narottamdas and Pushpaben who made Ayurvedic principles a way of life for me. To my gorgeous husband Raja whose love, support and guidance is unconditional. To my two daughters Shailu and Priti who work so hard alongside me and ensure all my ventures succeed. To my manageress Magda Reggio, who is like a daughter to me, and my good friends Cherie, Lyndsey and Gail Booth, Jane Goldsmith and my friends 'Toli': Thank you.

My gratitude goes to my dear friends at Thorsons, Eileen Campbell and Wanda Whiteley, for their continual belief in me and Caroline Shott at Alma Management, who after five years of working together has become a close friend and ally. Finally to the many journalists who continue to believe in my philosophies including Lorraine Kelly, Emma Moore, Lisa Aziz, Beverley d'Silva, Susan Clark, Kathy Philips, Karen Wheeler, Julia Carling, Lisa Podmore, Heather McGlone, Robina Dam, Vicky Wisdom, Janine Josman, Caroline Hogg, Caroline Hendrie, Arti Halai, Sawar and Sameena Ahmed, Yasmin Quereshi, Robert Norton at ClickMango, Sophie Fiennes, Michael van Stratton and John Gustavson.

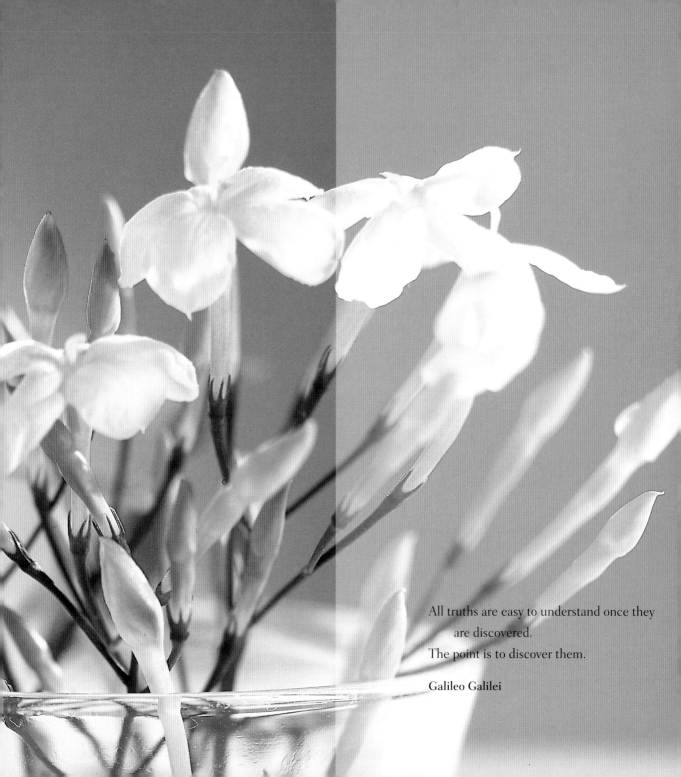

All truths are easy to understand once they
  are discovered.
The point is to discover them.

Galileo Galilei

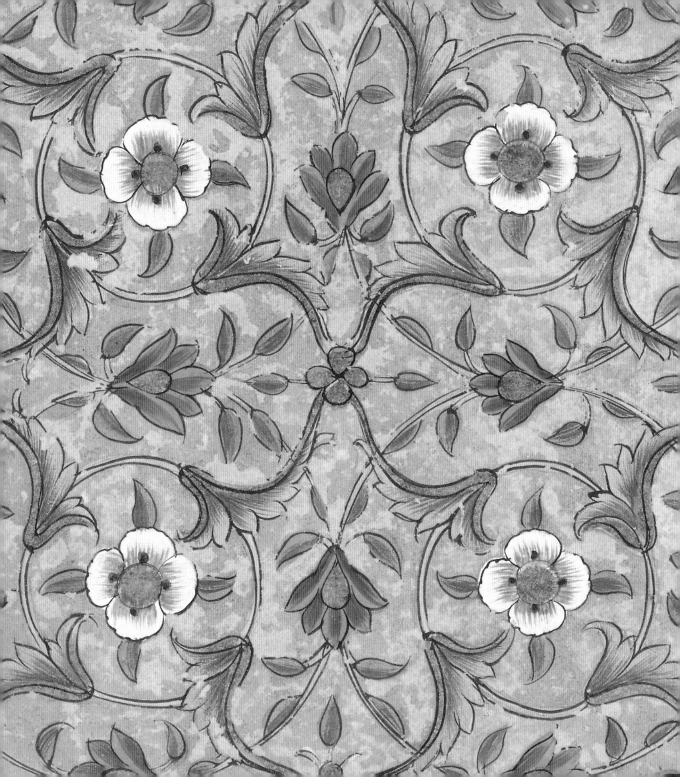

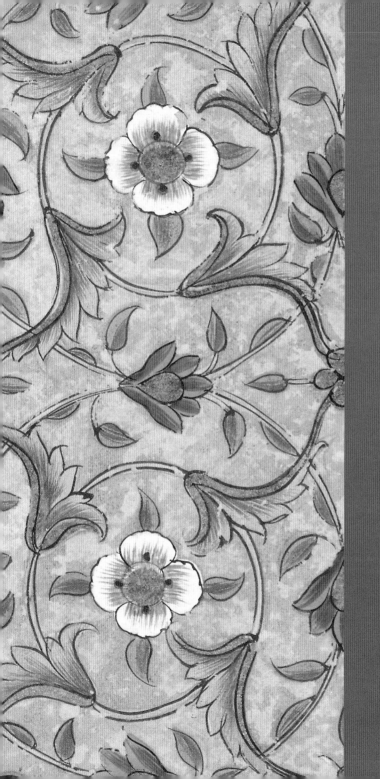

Ayurveda

The Science of Life

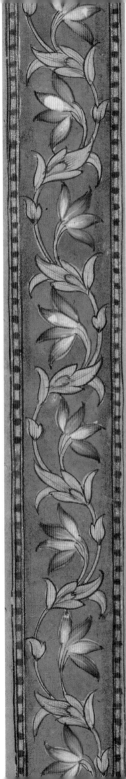

Introduction

My abiding philosophy is that beauty is not skin deep. In fact, my favourite mantra, practised daily in my London clinic, is, 'Beauty on the outside begins on the inside.' In this book we will go deeper in pursuit of this truism, drawing on the world's oldest medical system – Ayurveda – to show ways you can enhance your health and prolong your life. We will explore the realm of internal health and how crucial it is to maintaining that external twinkle in your eye, luminosity in your skin and, most important of all, the feeling of wellbeing that is so fundamental for real happiness. This book is concerned with giving you digestible insights that can be easily incorporated into your lifestyle.

The key to Ayurveda, India's most ancient holistic healing system, is in treating the mind, body and spirit as one entity to ensure total harmony and wellbeing. A treatment might entail oil therapy, yoga, meditation and massage, and what is so wonderful is that it is all natural. With our busy lifestyles, the new millennium is definitely the right time for Ayurveda.

Ayurveda translates literally as 'the science of life' and this holistic and most natural science exists in academic texts in a wealth of fascinating detail. Legend has it that three millennia ago a group of 52 Indian sages left their villages and travelled high into the Himalayas in search of enlightenment,

The key to Ayurveda is treating the mind,

with a particular altruistic brief: They wanted to learn how to eradicate disease from the world. Enlightenment could only occur to those fortunate few who were both physically and spiritually healthy, therefore they reasoned that to help other people to find true spiritual happiness they needed to find a way to free them from illness first.

The Rishis, as they were called, meditated collectively on solving this seemingly intractable dilemma. Eventually divine inspiration came when the nature of mental and physical health and happiness was revealed. The Rishis carefully preserved them in the ancient Vedic texts – documents which are the Hindu equivalent of the Bible. Since then, the secrets of health and happiness have been passed down from generation to generation. Today, Ayurveda remains the pre-eminent source of traditional medicine in India, Nepal and Sri Lanka.

In its rich historical texts, Ayurveda is a wonderfully complex practical and theoretical subject … and, until now, the preserve only of those with plenty of time to spend studying the theory. However, in this book I have done all the work for you, distilling the complexities of this vibrant, but intricate health regime into an easy-to-use, easy-to-understand simplified formula to which anyone can refer in order to bring the health elements, beauty know-how and home remedies of Ayurveda effortlessly into your life. Ayurveda functions on two levels, as a system of prevention for the woman or man keen to learn a holistic approach to self-care, and also as a medical science involving many years of study. This book should be read as a philosophy of health, not a medical text. I am a health facilitator and my focus is on easy-care preventative medicine. Therefore, throughout the text you will find sound and practical information that applies to aiding the health of every one of us. In addition, you will find specific detail that shows how you can further help your own body type by incorporating advice and know-how from this most traditional of all holistic therapies.

Ayurveda basics:

Ayurveda functions on two levels, as a system of prevention for the woman or man keen to learn a holistic approach to self-care, and also as a medical science involving many years of study.

body and spirit as one entity to ensure total harmony.

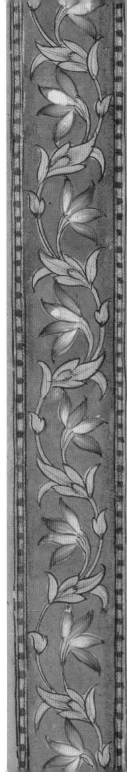

As well as having lots to say about improving poor health, Ayurveda is also the oldest example of the 'prevention is better than cure' philosophy. By treating the mind, body and spirit with herbal medicines, oil therapy, massage, yoga and meditation it is a system that aims to sustain health, rather than focusing purely on making ill people better. For the Ayurvedic sages believed that the pure health of every individual is their natural state, and any deviation is the sickness from which the Ayurvedic practitioner seeks to return his patient.

What this means for us in the West is that Ayurveda's focus on cleansing and purification (*Panchakarma*) and rejuvenation (*Rasayana*) is a great counterbalance to our stressed-out, polluted urban lives. In the West we are obsessed with making money, calorie-counting, staying slim and looking young. We relieve the stress all this creates by drinking alcohol, smoking and taking drugs, and then try and salvage our ravaged bodies with food supplements, quick trips to the health farm when we can afford them, expensive creams and facelifts, and a great deal of angst and frustration.

But Ayurveda views life in a more honest way. It teaches presentation and self-care. It stresses the importance of fuelling yourself with healthy food, exercising your body, offering your mind the tranquil spaces of meditation and finding solace in natural remedies – not chemical ones – during times when the body is temporarily out of balance. It is a wonderfully inspiring, common sense philosophy of listening to, understanding and interpreting what your body is saying to you.

The underlying philosophy is that it is not enough to treat just the symptoms of disease. Effective treatment encompasses the entire body.

Ayurveda makes a clear connection between emotional distress and physical deterioration. This holistic view suggests that illnesses affect mind and body and both should therefore be treated together. If you have a headache or back pain it is only natural that it will affect your mental well-being. Equally, your mood also feeds your state of health. Put simply, if you are depressed you are more prone to suffer physical complaints because you

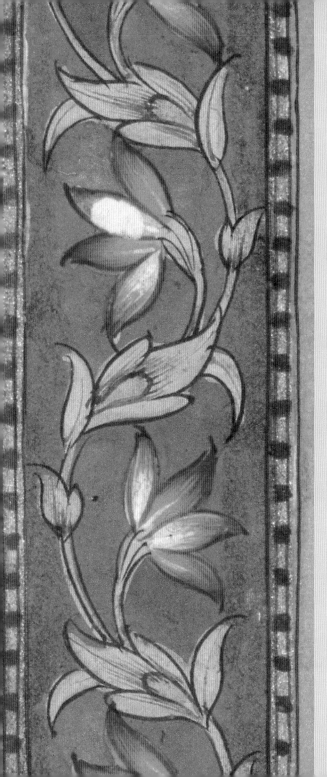

THE ideas and philosophies that underpin Ayurveda were cemented by the wise sages, or *Rishis*, of India more than 3000 years ago. They felt it necessary to remove themselves from the stress of daily living in order to meditate upon the diseases that afflict all creatures and prevent self-enlightenment. An inspired group of them gathered together in the foothills of the Himalayas and wrote down the insights that came to them. Some insights were said to be divinely inspired, others from their collective contemplation. These combined instructions – found in the best known Ayurvedic text, the *Charaka Samhita* – form the basis of modern Ayurveda.

will not care for yourself or eat as sensibly as you should. Conversely, if you are happy and buoyant you are much less likely to feel ill. An Ayurvedic healer does not just prescribe quick-fix herbs to treat illnesses, like Western doctors handing out antibiotics, but would instead supplement this with an entire change-of-lifestyle plan or revised eating suggestions at the very least. Strange, isn't it, that in the West we proudly label this approach complementary medicine, and hail the doctors who have the vision to practise it as visionary or cutting edge, when in fact they are sensibly following principles that are as old as the hills.

Ayurveda is a complete and balanced approach for creating and sustaining physical and mental harmony; the focus is upon the individual lifestyle, not upon the condition. It is clearly much more appropriate when trying to maintain health, assess illness and treat afflictions to view all elements of a person's lifestyle, diet, exercise routine, metabolism, body type and inherited characteristics as contributing parts of a larger whole. We do not exist in isolation. No man, or woman, is an island. Equally, no part of our mental, physical and spiritual system is separate from any other. The way we feel, what we eat, how much we exercise, how much stress we are under, what illnesses our parents suffered and so on, all determine our state of wellbeing.

Ayurvedic practitioners believe that an imbalance in one area of health can have a number of different causes depending on the background of the afflicted individual. The way this is done is through classification of everyone according to three fundamental types. At the heart of Ayurveda is the concept that there are three universal governing forces at work inside us all. These are called the *doshas* and they are described as Fire, Air and Earth. They are in a state of continual flux at work inside all of us, but there is a tendency for one or two to dominate in each person. You are created with an inborn doshic disposition that affects not only your physical characteristics – body shape, skin type, colouring and metabolism – but also your emotional and mental temperament. Your individual type (known as your '*prakriti*') can in

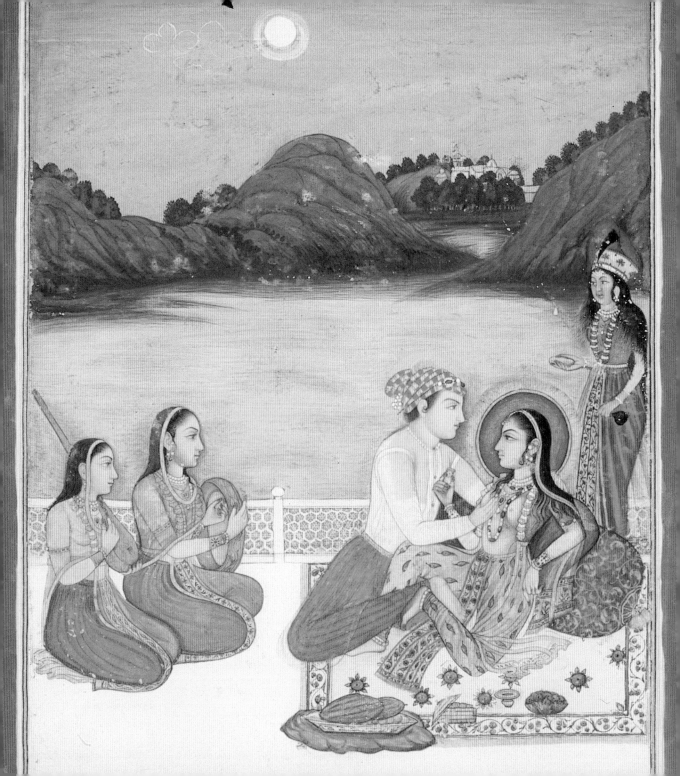

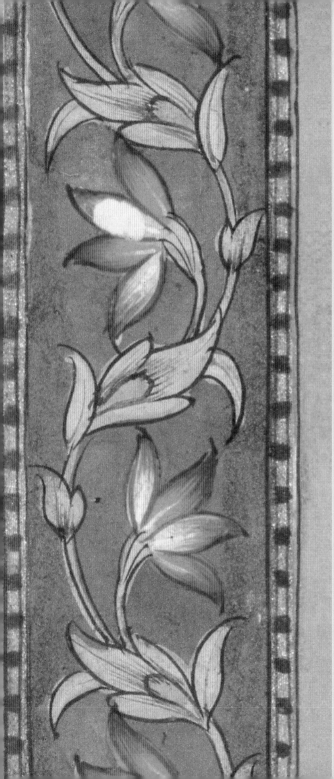

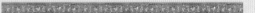

ACCORDING to Ayurveda, human beings consist of three components known as the physical, the subtle and the causal. In contemporary speech these equate to body, mind and spirit. Ayurveda believes that health flows from the balanced union of these three elements.

AYURVEDA is a Sanskrit word which comes from 'vid', meaning knowledge, and 'ayus', which means life cycle. It therefore represents a system of knowledge and advice about daily living, and for this reason is also known as 'the science of life'.

BLOOD-LETTING developed as part of traditional ancient Ayurveda. It was believed to stimulate the immune system and to eliminate toxins that might have accumulated in the deeper tissues.

turn give clues towards the type of illnesses from which you are most likely to suffer and help you begin to take steps to avoid them. For one of the fundamental principles of Ayurveda is that all illness is a result of disturbances in your doshic type. And although people with different doshic types may display similar symptoms, or attach the same label to their complaint or illness, appropriate treatment depends on the individual constitution or type.

It is this holistic emphasis that makes Ayurveda the ideal health philosophy for the new millennium. Although ancient, it could not be more relevant to the needs of today. Perhaps this is why it is the fastest growing lifestyle belief system after Buddhism, with increasing numbers of Western adherents embracing its commonsense and practical philosophies as a modus operandi for general health. But don't worry, it's not a religion. There is no belief system necessary, just sound commonsense mixed with an interest in ancient Indian wisdom and an open-minded approach to the herbal remedies, kitchen cupboard solutions and the yoga, massage and meditation approaches that Ayurveda advocates (none of which are necessary if they are simply not for you).

In the West we don't have time in our lives for a health regime that takes hours each day. That is why we have extracted the fundamentals for you, producing this handy but definitive Ayurveda lifestyle companion. Within it, we touch on ailments that can be helped using Ayurvedic practices, preventative medicine, yoga, massage, diet and beauty methods. Kept by your side, it will form an essential health manual that will give you a thorough understanding of Ayurveda in a practical light, showing how you can incorporate its techniques into the everyday lives of all the family.

This book takes a simple and practical look at how to use the principles of Ayurveda in your everyday health and beauty care. Thus with my down-to-earth approach you will be encouraged to adapt your own lifestyle and find out what's right for your type. The great thing is that if you choose not to follow the entire programme you can still gain fantastic benefits by picking and choosing the elements that enhance the way you choose to live your life.

Ayurveda basics:

Ayurveda identifies 107 points in an 'energy matrix' throughout the body throughout which 'prana' – the life force – flows. They are known as 'marmas' and are akin to the acupuncture points in Chinese medicine. Traditional Ayurvedic practitioners apply a combination of therapies, including herbal packs, massage and steam, at specific marma points to break down the blockages that they sense in their patient. The belief is that without this intervention the blockages will cause physical and mental symptoms, including bowel problems, skin complaints, anxiety, immune dysfunction, chronic fatigue and insomnia.

The History

Ayurveda basics:

It is this holistic emphasis that makes Ayurveda the ideal health philosophy for the new millennium.

Ayurveda originated in India and has been used extensively for more than 3000 years. It works on the principle of balance and prevention, and is a completely holistic approach to life. Ayurvedic practitioners believe that all parts of life (people, food, animals, nature, disease and the universe) are combinations of three energy elements: *Air* (vata), *Fire* (pitta) and *Earth* (kapha). Each person has a unique type, blueprint (or doshic mix), where one or two of these elements are more dominant. Which type you are depends on which of these elements are most prevalent. In general terms, Air (vata) types are creative, slender, highly strung types who are prone to suffer from insomnia and hate confrontation; Earth (kapha) types are large, slow-moving, placid, dislike change and must be careful with rich food in order to avoid piling on too much weight. Fire (pitta) types are ambitious, focused, of medium build and can be confrontational; they must be careful not to overdo the summer sun, arguments and spicy food. Tom Cruise and Nicole Kidman are both fast thinking creative types, but Nicole is Air-Fire and Tom is Air-Earth. Tony Blair is a stable Earth-Fire, but Cherie is a flightier Air-Earth. Posh Spice is Air-Earth, but David Beckham is a more irritable Fire-Earth type.

Ayurveda basics:

Ayurvedic practitioners believe that all parts of life (people, food, animals, nature, disease and the universe) are combinations of three energy elements: Air (vata), Fire (pitta) and Earth (kapha).

Illness is a deviation from your individual type; it occurs when your less dominant elements begin to take over your system, or your main element grows too strong. All disorders, therefore, are explained as excesses of one or more elements which need to be corrected. For depending on our type, Ayurveda says that each of us is at risk of developing specific health problems when we are under stress or suffering imbalance. For example, a Fire (pitta) imbalance can send ambition over the edge into

Ayurveda is a completely holistic approach to life

aggression, and impatience to rage. Earth types who become unbalanced tend to find their calm serenity transmuting into sulking and grumpiness, while an excess of Air sends enthusiasm racing over the edge into hyper-activity.

But remember that these pure single-type people are fairly uncommon. And even someone who is a fairly pure Air, Fire or Earth type will still exhibit some attributes of the other doshas from time to time. For example an Air type who starts piling on the pounds is suffering the effects of too much Earth (kapha) influence. A placid Earth type who spends a week feeling irritable and snappish is experiencing an over-abundance of Fire (pitta). What you need to do then is eat foods or use herbal remedies that re-energize your core again. Generally speaking, however, you need to stock up on the elements that your mind and body lack, so you do not over-reinforce your natural type. Thus if you are Air (vata) you will become over-animated and stressed out if you don't bring some moderating Earth and Fire elements into your constitution. More on this later.

Ayurveda basics:

Illness is a deviation from your individual type, it occurs when your less dominant elements begin to take over your system, or your main element grows too strong.

13

S i m p l y

A y u r v e d a

THE Ayurvedic creation myth suggests that in the beginning there was nothing but pure consciousness. There was nothing to see, touch or hear. But then the vibrations of the first sound began. This led to the creation of the first element, Ether. When this began to move a breeze began to blow and Air was created. In time, the movement of the Ether produced friction which led to Heat. Light came from the Heat and eventually Fire was created. This warmth helped to dissolve parts of the Ether which became Water. When this solidified it became Earth.

and works on the principle of prevention and balance.

Ayurvedic Influence upon Bharti's Childhood

I grew up in Kenya, the daughter of Indian parents, before coming to Britain as an adult. As a child, Ayurveda was a fundamental part of life as it is for millions of Indian families around the world. My parents were compounders, the early pharmacists, who would mix whatever the doctors had prescribed, but although they were dealing with modern chemicals, they retained their interest in herbal remedies which we also used regularly at home. My grandfather, who died before I was born, was an Ayurvedic doctor. This meant my father grew up immersed in an Ayurvedic culture which ran alongside his Western pharmaceutical training. A source of great fascination when I was young was his little cabinet full of a fascinating and colourful array of powered herbs. Whenever we were ill he would go into his box, and mix a little of this with a little of that. We thought he was just making it up and would giggle when he would emerge and present, with a flourish, a small packet of herbal powder and tell us to take it three times a day. I'm sure that some of his potions we regarded rather disparagingly, just as Western children regard cod liver oil.

Ayurveda informed my childhood, even though I was not aware of it at the time. If I had a headache, my parents would always look knowingly at me and then pronounce, 'We can see the headache in your eyes' – according to Ayurveda the eyes are the first area of the body affected by a headache. Whenever I had a sore throat and would be almost losing my voice, my parents responded by mixing milk with turmeric – one of the most potent healing Ayurvedic herbs – and adding a little dab of butter 'to coat the inside

Ayurveda basics:

Each person has a unique type, blueprint (or doshic mix), where one or two of the three elements are more dominant.

'Daughter, if I am not here tomorrow,

TRADITIONAL Ayurveda suggests three most unusual causes of disease which provide a fascinating insight into the climate in which the system was developed 3000 years ago:

MISUSE OF THE MIND AND BODY – this included overindulgence in sexual activity, immodest behaviour, lack of respect for one's elders, anger, fear, vanity, greed, hatred, lies and disregard of local customs.

UNHEALTHY ASSOCIATION OF THE SENSE ORGANS – this included over or under stimulation of the sense organs, very unpleasant odours, gazing upon things that are alarming or unattractive.

VAGARIES OF TIME AND SEASON – this included daytime sleep when not prescribed, vigorous exercise after sunset, disregard for natural cycles.

of your throat'. Of course at the time it wasn't explained to us that this remedy was steeped in history, we were simply told to take it and of course, being children, we hated it.

As a family we would fast on the first Monday of each month. As I grew older I began to see the sense in this. Ayurveda is a way of disciplining and calming down your digestive system. Your system gets very mixed up if you

Ayurveda basics:

In Ayurveda all disorders, can be explained as excesses of one or more elements.

learn this from me while I am alive.'

indulge in food at all hours of the day. That is why, according to strict Ayurvedic thinking, it is better for your constitution and general health to try and stick to regular mealtimes. When I started training as a beauty therapist I met an old man, the father of a friend of my husband, who was a great believer in Ayurvedic herbalism. He was more than one hundred years old and still taking daily walks. No-one would think he was that age. He was an inquisitive fellow with a young heart and one day he said to me, 'I understand you are studying beauty therapy, tell me about it.' So I told him that in the Western world it is important to look and feel good all the time. He contemplated what I had said, before responding with the words: 'Daughter, if I am not here tomorrow, learn this from me while I am alive. If you want anybody's skin to be nice and clear, if you do not clear their gut and their lungs they will never have healthy skin.' What he was telling me was pure Ayurvedic teaching. Your body is composed of what you eat, so if your gut is congested eventually the system starts failing. We find that most of the people who visit our clinic in London are constipated. They do not drink enough water. It makes perfect sense that if you are not eliminating waste food products how can your mouth be ready to eat? You need to wait and let the system clear itself before continuing to feed. In the meantime you should drink copious quantities of water to flush out your body. My father-in-law is 86 years old and lives with my husband and I. He has always practised Ayurveda, and its system underpins his life. If he has constipation he will stop eating. He says simply: 'Until the other system opens I'm not letting any more food inside.'

When the influence of Western medicine first arrived in India and Kenya, people forgot about their herbal remedies, but only for a short time. Now, when you go to India and listen to people ordering items in their local pharmacy, first and foremost you hear them ask for Ayurvedic preparations. And now, in America and in Britain we are seeing the rise and rise of the Ayurveda system of health as it becomes increasingly fashionable.

The Ayurvedic Dosha Questionnaire

The first step towards benefiting from Ayurveda is to determine your body type or dosha, so you can apply specific information in the book. Everyone is different, but Ayurveda believes there are three broad brush-strokes. Each individual is controlled by these three elements to varying degrees, but we usually have one or possibly two dominant doshas. Which mixture of types you are (known as your '*prakriti*') is determined by your behavioural traits as well as body size and composition, food preferences, energy levels, and metabolism. Discovering your type is the most significant step in finding out more about how Ayurveda can be helpful to you.

The easiest way to find out which sections of this book will have most meaning for you and your friends and family is to take the following lifestyle questionnaire. Circle the statement that applies most.

Physical assessment:

A   I am slim and fine-boned with only soft muscular definition
B   I am of medium physique with fairly good muscular development
C   I am of large build, prone to roundness and gain weight easily

A   I can eat what I want without having to worry about putting on weight
B   I gain weight if I eat too much, but can lose it if I try
C   If I put on weight, which I do fairly easily, it's a real struggle to shed it

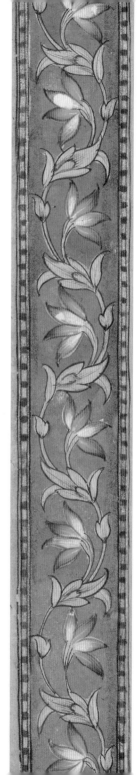

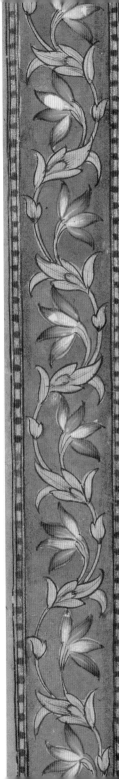

A   My skin is cool, rough and prone to being quite dry in places

B   My skin is warm and prone to oiliness

C   My skin is smooth, cool to the touch and hardly ever dry

A   My underlying skin tone is best described as bluish

B   My underlying skin tone is best described as reddish

C   My underlying skin tone is best described as yellowish

A   My skin is prone to dehydration and dryness, especially when it is cold outside

B   I suffer rashes and inflammation and sometimes burn

C   I sometimes suffer from whiteheads and blackheads

A   My complexion is marked by fine lines and prominent veins

B   I have some broken capillaries, freckles and moles

C   My skin is supple and soft

A   My hair has a natural curl and can be quite dry on the ends

B   My hair is fairly straight and fine

C   My hair is wavy, thick and lustrous

A   My eyes are small and pale, dark brown, grey or slate blue

B   My eyes are bright blue, light brown, lustrous and bright

C   My eyes are large, liquidic and brown

A   My lips are dry and quite slender

B   I have fairly average soft red lips

C   My lips are firm, large and quite plump

A   My fingernails are quite dry, brittle and can be rough

B   I have soft pink fingernails that don't split often

C   My fingernails are thick, smooth and very strong

Physical tendencies

A   I prefer warm weather to cold

B   I prefer cool weather and particularly enjoy cold foods like ice-cream and ice cold drinks

C   I enjoy most climates but prefer warmer weather

A   My energy is inconsistent and usually comes in bursts

B   My energy levels are moderate

C   My energy tends to be fairly steady when apparent but I'm often lazy

A   I am active but I lose strength quickly

B   I enjoy physical activity and sweat easily

C   I have good endurance but I'm naturally lethargic

A   I am active and restless, and what I lack in strength I make up for in enthusiasm

B   I have average stamina and good staying power

C   I have very good stamina and physical endurance

A   I do not usually require much sleep and I sleep lightly

B   I need a moderate amount of sleep and sleep soundly

C   I enjoy sleep and sleep deeply

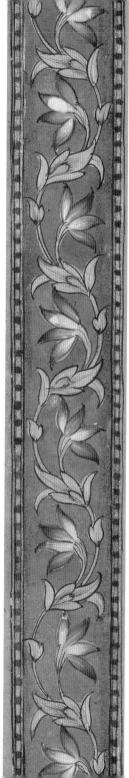

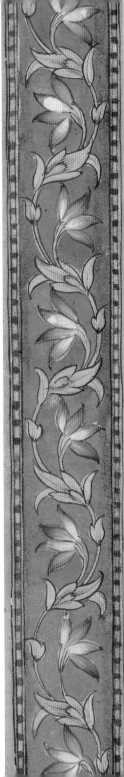

A I am talkative and tend to talk quite fast

B I have a fairly confident voice and can be an assertive speaker

C I have a gentle voice and talk fairly slowly

A My appetite is irregular, I eat what I want when I want it

B I have a good appetite and tend to eat regularly

C I eat fairly slowly, enjoy food and have a consistently good appetite

A My elimination is irregular and I am prone to constipation

B My elimination is fairly regular

C I am rarely constipated

A I alternate between dry and loose stools

B I have soft stools that tend to be loose

C Food moves through me slowly

A I sometimes experience low appetite, low back pain and muscle spasms

B I can suffer with hot flushes, acid stomach and heartburn

C I have trouble with sinus congestion, coughs, colds, and weight gain

Temperament assessment

A I learn new things easily, but I tend to forget easily as well

B My memory is good

C Although I tend to learn slowly, I go on to have good recall

A I tend to be enthusiastic and vivacious with an active imagination

B I tend to be somewhat orderly and precise and can be easily irritated

C I am steady, calm and infrequently ruffled

A When I am stressed I suffer anxiety attacks, insomnia and sometimes hysteria

B Under stress I can become jealous, hostile, frustrated and easy to anger

C If I am under too much pressure I become depressed, despondent and possessive

A I am upset by buffeting winds and cold

B Heat and sun make me edgy

C When it is cold and damp I feel miserable

A My moods fluctuate, often fairly unpredictably

B I am goal and task driven, my moods are a secondary consideration

C I am consistently compassionate and caring

A I am creative and imaginative, I like to express myself

B I am a perfectionist who likes to be organized and efficient

C My thoughts and ideas are well organized and tend to be fairly tranquil

A My thoughts are often dreams which I do not need to see through to their conclusion

B My ideas and thoughts tend to be well-considered and logical

C I am thorough and good at following through

A I choose an unpredictable, exciting lifestyle and hate routine

B I like my life to be busy but wouldn't say I hate routine

C I enjoy a relaxed and fairly slow-paced routine lifestyle

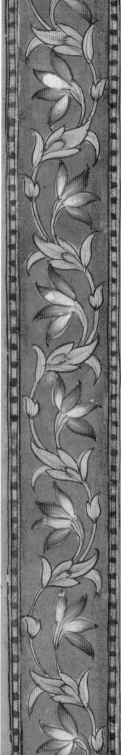

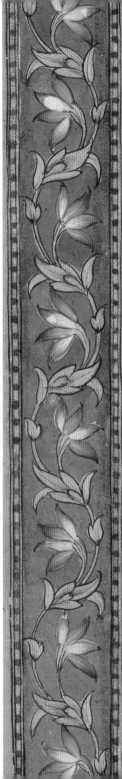

Results:

Mostly As: **Air** (vata) type – You are a natural whirlwind, always on the go and as energetic and unpredictable as your type name suggests. You are artistic and tender, but can be over-sensitive and prone to burnout when you don't take enough time to care for yourself or try to cram too much into every week. You can be visionary and at your best you are highly creative and imaginative – at whatever you choose to put your mind to, but when you overload yourself you experience digestive problems, you get scatty, prone to sensitive dry skin, sleepless nights and you become less effective. You need to avoid the crash-and-burn option by making time to chill out and, however loathsome it may sound, trying to coax a few more elements of routine into your life. Try Tai Chi, walking, dancing, yoga, or, when you feel yourself getting overwrought, make a few days space to chill out and unwind.

Airy types include Gwyneth Paltrow, Leonardo DiCaprio and Julia Roberts.

Mostly Bs: **Fire** (pitta) type. You are one of life's alchemists, blazing a trail, making a difference, taking no prisoners. You are as fiery and passionate as your type name suggests, dynamic, active and inspirational. There is never a dull minute around you. When your life is in balance you have the attractive commanding presence of the natural leader, you radiate perception and focus, and love taking control and encouraging other people to have a good time. But if you overdo it, don't fuel your body with the right foods and give in to your more fiery excesses, you can become brittle, critical, overly competitive, and your skin can flare up as a visual indication of your internal combustion. You need to cool down, controlling the excesses of your inflamed inner core – think fun exercise like skiing, swimming and cycling to give the physical expression you require without bombarding yourself within an environment of competitiveness. Take a breath before you respond, learn the art of compromise, and make enough time to relax.

Fiery types include Jennifer Aniston, Marco Pierre White and Cindy Crawford.

Mostly Cs: **Earth** (kapha) type. At your best you are as deliciously grounded and dependable as your type name suggests. You are solid, patient and intensely loyal. You are drawn towards people, who are in turn drawn to confide in you, and are a wonderful source of constancy and solidity in a crisis. But when out of balance that laid-back charm can turn into excess sluggishness and your skin can become excessively oily. If you don't ensure that enough is going on you tend to vegetate, seeking solace in the third bar of chocolate and feeling a bit stagnant internally. If you feel this happening you need to act fast, and top up your self-esteem and energy levels with plenty of fresh fruit and vegetables. You have fantastic endurance and would really benefit from running, tennis and aerobics, all sports that get your metabolism moving.

Grounded types include Oprah Winfrey, Kate Winslet and Dawn French.

Mixed Types

If you scored fairly evenly across two types you are a combination type. Most people are a double type (two doshas present in high proportions) but one type will tend to be dominant. This one is always named first and is considered the leading dosha. So if you scored highly in Air and Fire, but had marginally more points for Fire, you are a Fire-Air type and your dominant type is Fire. You can benefit from reading both your type sections. Follow the daily routine and seasonal lifestyle recommendations for your most dominant type, but read the advice for both your doshas. So if you are Earth-Air you should follow an Air reducing diet in late fall and early winter, and an Earth reducing diet in spring and early summer.

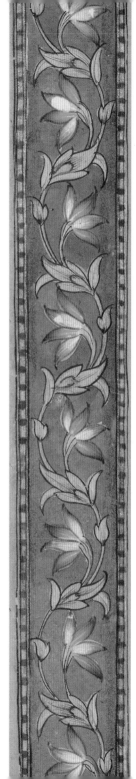

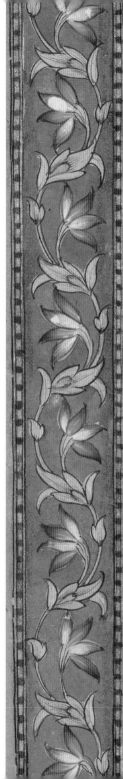

A much smaller percentage of people are what is called a tridosha type, meaning they scored almost equally across all three types. This is an unusual blessing and means you are said to face a long and happy life with few problems. If you should score fairly evenly across all three types, it might be prudent to read the descriptions above and pick the type that best describes you.

Understanding Health Problems

Before you can correct physical health problems it helps to understand what is causing them. If you are suffering from an excess of one of the doshas – and anyone can experience the ill effects of being overloaded with the effects of too much Air, Earth or Fire, whatever their type – evaluating your symptoms is a very useful way of discovering the balance of influences in your body. You are most likely to experience symptoms of aggravation of your own type, but anyone can end up with a dosha imbalance.

Typical symptoms of aggravated Air in all types:

Air is particularly active in the heart, colon, bones, thighs, ears, skin, brain, nervous system, bladder, lungs and pelvis.
Air is in charge of all motion in the body and the mind.

Too much Air leads to problems including the separation of tissue – such as dry flaking skin; increased movement – such as diarrhoea; decreased movement – such as cramps or pins and needles; unusual movement – such as tremors or twitches.

Typical symptoms of aggravated Fire in all types:

Fire is in charge of all processes of transformation in the body.

Fire is particularly active in the spleen, small intestine, brain, liver, skin, eyes, endocrine glands, blood and sweat.

Too much Fire leads to problems including inflammations, fever, burning rashes and over-sensitive skin, hyperacidity, indigestion, hot or burning diarrhoea, ulcerations and anaemia.

Typical symptoms of aggravated Earth in all types:

Earth is the stabilizing influence in the body and mind, it calms, lubricates and maintains the system.

Earth is particularly active in the head and neck, stomach, lungs, heart, lymph, joints, brain, mouth and fat.

Too much Earth leads to problems including excessive production of mucus, itchy skin, a pallid complexion, difficulty breathing, heaviness and lethargy of mind and spirit.

Seasonal Routines

There are three seasons in the Ayurvedic calendar – winter, spring and summer. Your body – whatever your type – changes with the weather that each season brings.

Spring: Crisp windy weather increases **Air**
Summer: Hot weather increases **Fire**
Winter: Cold wet weather increases **Earth**

If the dosha increases too much you can find your body out of balance. Therefore, with the changing seasons you need to balance your body's natural predisposition to fluctuate or you might find yourself out of balance. Along with each description of type below you will therefore find simple guidelines on how best to care for yourself as the year wheels around.

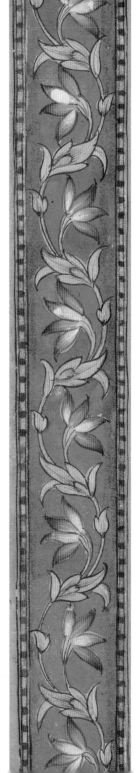

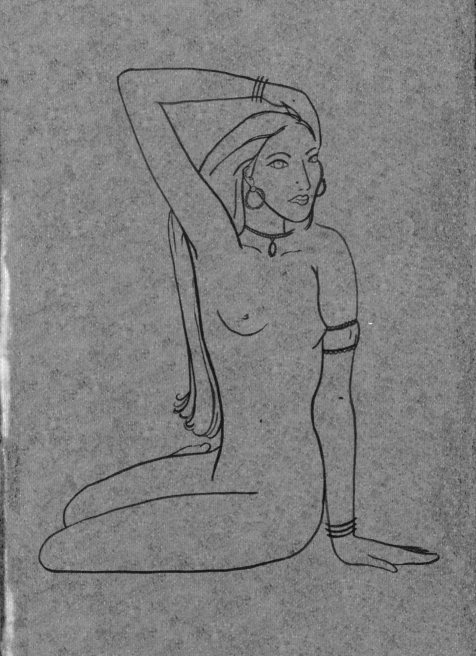

Air is characterized by boundless

Air (Vata)

Temperament

Ethereal and creative, pure Air-dominant types can also be unreliable, nervous and changeable, darting from one thing to another, but often displaying striking originality of thought, bursts of lateral thinking and admirable decisiveness. Memory can be poor; although quick to learn they often do not retain new knowledge. The media is full of airy types, they are attracted by the vibrancy, immediacy and constant stimulation of close access to new information. The flip side is that they can suffer from insomnia, can be restless if not occupied and more than any other type are prone to depression, tension and worries. Money flows in ... and out again. They are characterized by boundless reserves of energy, both physical and nervous, and by their vivaciousness. These are active, quick people who always seem to be on the move. They frequently have an interest in spirituality and those with psychic abilities seem to be more common among this type than any other. When they dream they are participants in a dynamic, active symbolic world of flying, running, climbing and jumping.

Physique

Air-dominant types tend to be slender, light in weight – even insubstantial and bony – and do not gain weight very easily. But they are usually either very tall or very short. When young, they are usually amongst the most athletic in

Air basics:

Air are active, quick people who always seem to be on the move.

reserves of energy, both physical and nervous.

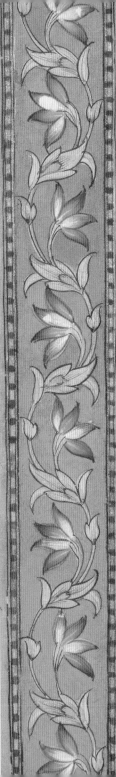

the class, but tend not to have excessive muscle mass. They can have small-ish eyes, fairly fine hair and delicate eyelashes.

Other features

If you are Air-dominant, you are probably used to dealing with dry skin, your voice may be pitched high and light, and you may be prone to biting your fingernails. You tend to eat quickly, enjoy your food and do not worship regular meal times. You do not eliminate copiously and may suffer constipation. You probably have a fairly high sex drive and a fast, irregular heart-beat.

Typical daily routine to balance Air types:

Wake up: 30 minutes before sun rise.

Breakfast: Cooked cereal.

Teeth ritual: After you have brushed your teeth, massage your gums with triphala and sesame oil.

Gargling: Gargle with triphala tea (steep half a teaspoon in a cup) and chew three teaspoonfuls of black sesame seeds.

Favoured drink: Warm water with honey and lemon juice.

Bath/shower routine: Massage with sesame oil before bathing. Add a few drops of essential oil – jasmine or geranium – to your bath. Follow with an application of the massage oil recommended for your type.

Face care: Follow cleansing, nourishing and moisturizing routine.

Meditation suggestions: 20 minutes using the mantra for your type.

Lunch: Choose from the Air pacifying diet. Try to lie down for 15 minutes after eating with eyes closed.

Yoga practice: Alternate nostril breathing, sun salutation and the other postures recommended for your type.

Dinner: Eat around 7.30–8.30pm choosing food appropriate to your type.

Sunset suggestions: Wash your body and put on loose clean clothes before spending 20 minutes in meditation.

Night time ritual: Follow cleansing, nourishing and moisturizing routine for your skin type. Massage your scalp and feet with brahmi oil.

Sleep time: Try to turn your light out between 10–11pm.

Air case history 1

Bill, 42, is a signwriter. Deeply creative, responsive and changeable, he is a lateral thinker always searching for a career path that will catch his attention sufficiently. He has fed himself with various options, none of which seem to satisfy entirely. In the past 20 years he has worked as a journalist, motorcycle courier, environmentalist, graphic artist, oil painter, and even as a neon-glass bender. When he needs money he has the skills and attitude to simply get it pouring in, then all of a sudden he is off on a jaunt around the world, deeply immersed in the culture in which he is living. He returns enraptured until another inspiration strikes. He eats with great rapidity and has a visible excess of nervous energy, but however much he eats he never seems to put on weight. When a project captures his attention he devotes himself to his new passion, often staying up night after night to continue with his new, all-consuming interest. He is very popular with women, who are drawn to his complex, intriguing, quick-witted personality. His sexuality is capricious – he is either highly-sexed or completely disinterested in intimacy, often for months at a time. He has small, bright eyes that are always scanning the horizon for something to engage his attention. His hair is thinning and he is 5'9" tall, with slender limbs, a well-developed chest and a small waist and hips. He describes himself as: 'Always wanting to try something new.'

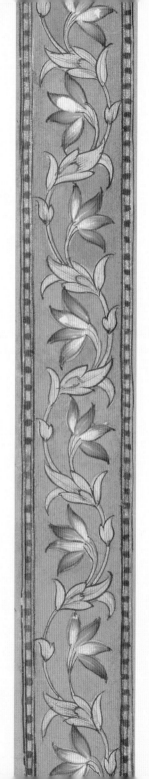

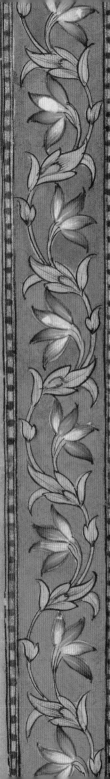

Seasonal lifestyle recommendations for Air types

In late autumn and through the winter you should eat plenty of warm, nourishing and fairly heavy grounding food and allow yourself more oil than during the rest of the year. Drink lots of hot drinks and avoid eating dry or uncooked foods, especially salads and raw vegetables, as they will excacerbate your chilly feelings. You can also indulge yourself by eating more sweet and sour and salty tastes, but try to steer clear of bitter, astringent and pungent food.

Typical health problems: Irritable bowel syndrome (especially among men), disorders of the nervous system, tension and anxiety, migraine, depression, heart problems, hypertension, constipation, insomnia, giddiness.

Air lifestyle checklist:

1. Try and meditate – or at least spend time in quiet contemplation – every day.
2. Avoid excessive physical activity, balance your energy and enthusiasm with sufficient rest and recuperation to sustain it.
3. Eat warm food and avoid very cold or frozen food.
4. Choose sweet, acid and salty food.
5. Avoid spicy and hot food, and do not eat too many nuts and seeds.
6. Avoid eating too many Air foods and stick to Earth and Fire foods instead.
7. Try and find a way to arrange regular massages to help you unwind and relax.
8. Go to bed early to encourage yourself to have enough time to calm down before sleep.

Air case history 2

Penny, 30, works as a reporter on a newspaper. She has seemingly boundless energy, is passionate about issues that move her, is warm-hearted, highly creative and decisive, but prone to sleepless nights worrying about tensions in her life. She believes that pushing energy into situations is the way to solve them, but can suffer from feelings of anxiety when under stress or in a confrontational situation. She has a slender frame, delicate bone structure, is 5'9" tall and weighs just over nine-and-a-half stone. In her free time Penny writes stories and paints murals. Her friends appreciate the energy and enthusiasm with which she invests every area of her life, and are also drawn to the air of mysticism that seems to surround her like a veil. She does nothing by halves, and can often go without much sleep until suddenly she is exhausted and needs a day or two in bed to recharge – after which time she is quickly bored of rest. She enjoys exotic food, but often forgets to eat when alone and can choose a poor, but convenient diet. She also has a history of biting her fingernails. She is always immersed in one project or another, and other more sedentary types often wonder how she manages to get so much done. She is interested in psychology and spirituality, but she is more motivated to gain an overview of a subject rather than taking the time to learn about a lesser amount in more detail, and her memory can be rather sketchy and unspecific. She describes herself as: 'Someone who is passionate about life and keen to know what is happening beneath the surface.'

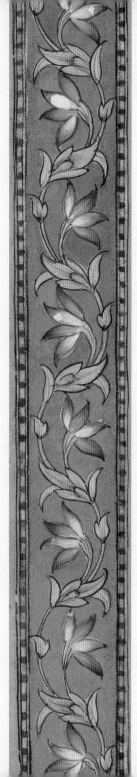

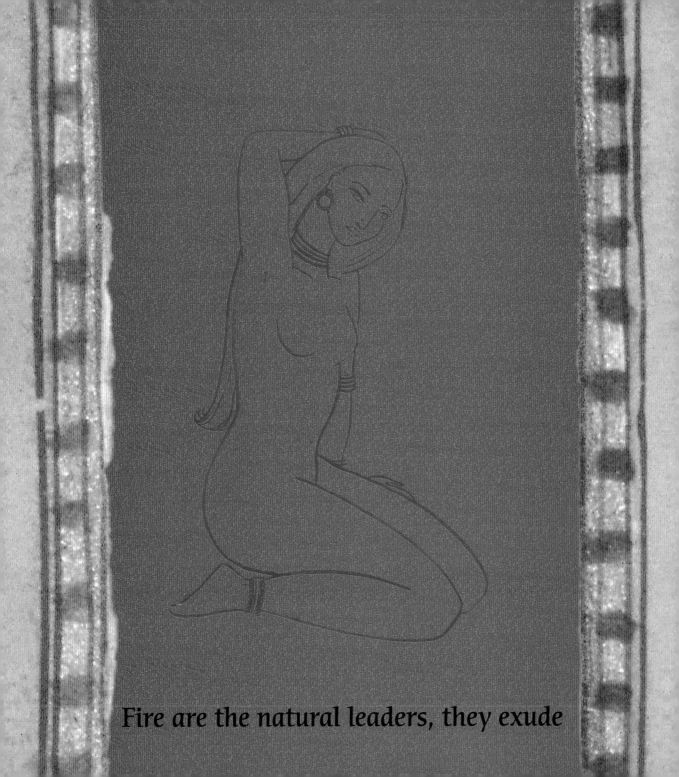

Fire are the natural leaders, they exude

Fire (Pitta)

Temperament

A Fire personality is much more stable than their type name suggests. In fact, they tend to be the most stable of all types, looking at life in a clear and rational way and are able to be wonderfully decisive when necessary. These are the natural leaders, they exude wisdom and consequently others are drawn to them for guidance. They are rational, sharp, ambitious and filled with direction, focus and common-sense. They live comfortably – neither frugally nor excessively – for theirs tend to be lives of balance. They are fairly active, but prefer to use their heads rather than their bodies when they work hard. They are open to new ideas, and sometimes might seem like logical cold fish, but inside their hearts beat warmly for those they respect and admire. They are the least showy of the types, have high intelligence but can be brittle when under stress, and when pushed can be judgmental, swiftly snap and become angry. They are often interested in sport, politics and science.

Physique

They can look older than their years. They are neither prone to carry excess weight nor to be skinny, but instead they are of medium build and average height, with smooth skin – often with freckles or moles.

Fire basics:

Fire are fairly active, but prefer to use their heads rather than their bodies when they work hard.

wisdom and other types are drawn to them.

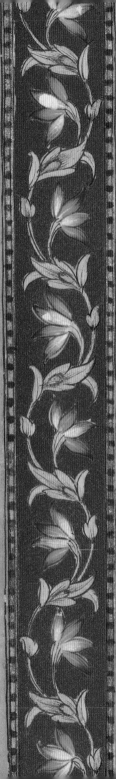

Other features

They tend to go grey early, and fiery men can go bald prematurely. They enjoy food, tend to eat sensibly and burn off calories efficiently. They are particularly drawn to bitter, astringent and sweet flavours, and they usually love cold drinks. They perspire freely, have hands that feel warm to the touch and dislike too much heat. Fire types need to urinate frequently and have loose stools and a tendency to diarrhoea.

Typical daily routine for Fire types

Wake up: An hour before sun rise.

Breakfast: Cold cereal.

Teeth ritual: After you have brushed your teeth, massage your gums with cardamom, a pinch of rock salt and sesame oil.

Gargling: Gargle with fennel or licorice tea (steep half a teaspoon in a cup) and chew two teaspoonfuls of black sesame seeds.

Morning drink: A quarter of a cup of aloe vera juice.

Bath/shower routine: Massage with coconut oil before bathing. Add a few drops of essential oil – sandalwood or vetiver – to your bath. Follow with an application of the massage oil recommended for your type.

Face care: Follow cleansing, nourishing and moisturizing routine.

Meditation suggestions: Practise cool breaths and spend 20 minutes in meditation using the mantra recommended for your type.

Lunch: Choose from the Fire pacifying diet. Try to lie down for 15 minutes after eating with eyes closed.

Yoga practice: Alternate nostril breathing, and the other postures recommended for your type.

Dinner: Eat arond 7.30–8.30pm choosing food appropriate to your type.

Sunset suggestions: Wash your body and put on loose clean clothes before spending 20 minutes in meditation.

Night time ritual: Follow cleansing, nourishing and moisturizing routine for your skin type. Massage your scalp and feet with brahmi oil.

Sleep time: Try to turn your light out between 10–11pm.

Typical health problems: Headaches, gall bladder and liver problems, digestive problems, skin complaints, jaundice, insomnia, excessive thirst.

Fire case history 1

Michael, 27, is a computer consultant who thrives on a fast-paced city lifestyle. He is ambitious, hard-working, intensely focused upon his work, and enjoys bringing the theoretical and abstract into a usable form. He reads avidly, can be cynical, laughs often, enjoys intellectual argument, and claims to need only four hours sleep a night. He has soft pale skin and prefers the air-conditioned environment where he works to the temperature variations of the outdoor world, and in the past five years has shown little inclination to exercise his body, although he used to play rugby and tennis at school. He says he prefers a good workout with a book. He began losing his hair prematurely several years ago, but isn't too concerned about his looks. He enjoys a good debate and holds tightly onto his real feelings. He is a private man who can appear superficially to be rather cold, but his modesty belies a commitment to those to whom he is close and who have earned his respect. He is of medium height and build, 5'9" tall, weighing 11 stone. His hands often feel clammy. He enjoys experimenting with exotic food and particularly enjoys the sweet and sour nature of Chinese dishes. He says of himself: 'I don't really mind what people think of me, I look for self-satisfaction and stimulation instead.'

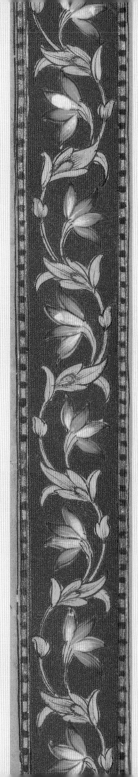

Fire case history 2

Charlotte, 55, is a food historian. She is a great entertainer and enjoys the art and craft of being a hostess. She is very warm to those in her inner circle, but maintains a certain reserve with those she does not know well, although she is always charming. She likes living well, but is never profligate or excessive in her attitude. She tends to choose some-what carefully and believes in the mantra of 'making do' – hoarding items that might come in useful one day. She is fairly conformist and traditional in her outlook, has a dry, witty and quick sense of humour, and well-considered and passionate intellectual opinions, but she is a powerhouse of strength for those close to her who are in need. She is a great organizer and is extremely methodical and forthright. She does not tolerate fools well, and when others exhibit muddle-headed or woolly thinking can become very judgmental, outspoken and critical. She is interested in history, music, technology and likes gentle gardening with a glass of wine in her hand. She is more interested in the genus of species than hard spade-work, and is involved with many historical and horticultural societies. Recently she began learning the clavichord. She does not like central heating, preferring to pull on a jumper and leave her windows open. She is 5'5" tall, weighs 8 stone and has soft pale skin covered in freckles. She says of herself: 'I thrive on intellectual stimulation and wit.'

Fire lifestyle checklist

1. Avoid exposing the body to too much sun.
2. Avoid excessive tea and coffee, salt and alcohol.
3. Expose your body to a cooling environment – take cooling baths rather than hot ones and go for walks after the sun has gone down.
4. Drink plenty of liquid, preferably lots of long cold drinks.
5. Avoid fizzy or acidic drinks and do not drink too much fruit juice.
6. Eat as many raw, cold foods, such as salad and fruit, as possible.
7. Choose bitter, astringent and sweet food.
8. Avoid eating Fire foods; instead, choose Air and Earth foods.

Seasonal lifestyle recommendations for Fire types

If you don't feel hungry in the summer go with this feeling. When you do eat stick to cooling food and drink so your digestive fire does not inflame you during your vulnerable season. The worst thing you could do is live on a diet of spicy curries! Far better to eat sweet, bitter foods and drink plenty of liquids. Avoid drinking ice cold drinks with your food as this can inhibit your digestive fire.

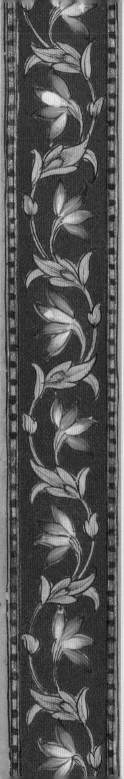

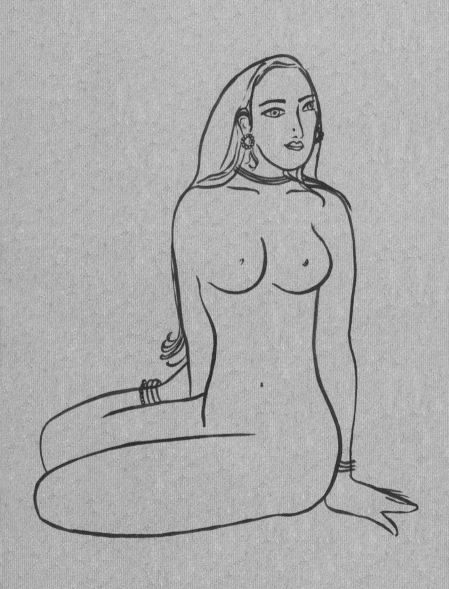

Earth types are the providers and nurturers.

Earth (Kapha)

Temperament

These are the junoesque earth mothers and well-padded pub regulars who are known for their calm, easy-going temperaments, warmth and jolly bonhomie. They are the most forgiving of all the types, placid, slow to anger or get excited, but sometimes equally slow to absorb new information, tending to trust tried and tested approaches over the more innovative. Earth dominant types move slowly and decisively, and tend to prefer more sedentary activities to more profound physical exertion. They can be masters of the art of getting other people to do things for them, but when necessary can rise to the challenge and cope well with hard physical labour especially when interests like gardens or their loved ones are involved. Earthy people are the providers, the nurturers of body and appetite, who create homely spaces and tend to people's physical and material needs as acts of devotion and concern. They sleep soundly and deeply, tend to snore and have to guard against spending too long in slumber, so enamoured are they are the comforts of their bedrooms. They tend to be resistant to change, enjoying tradition and believing that things tend to be better if they stay as they are. They are the stalwarts of local societies, rather than innovators. More materialistic than spiritual, they are the great conservationists – of money, energy and strength – and are easy to be around.

Earth basics:

Earth dominant types move slowly and decisively, and tend to prefer more sedentary activities to more profound physical exertion.

They are placid and the most forgiving of all types.

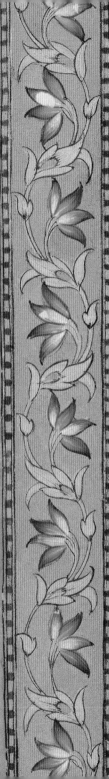

Earth case history 1

Jacqueline, 55, is a home-maker. She is very home-loving, protective and nurturing of her grown children; when they were younger she self-lessly devoted herself to their welfare. She is a people lover who is tactile and enjoys the warmth of physical contact. Her interests include country pursuits, the royal family, children and babies, horses, interior decorating, reading and art. She has a somewhat cautious approach to life in her mid-years, having been more adventurous when young. At the age of twenty, a doctor who treated her in the middle of the night for dysentery asked if she would forgive him an observation. She nodded and he suggested that she would grow up to be 'fat, fertile and flatulent'. She laughingly admits that this has mostly come true. She moves carefully now she is older and says experience has shown her it can be painful to fall. She never wanted a formal career, her guiding motivation was always to marry and have children. She has big bones, wide shoulders, is 5'6" tall and weighs 13 stone. She's been on more diets than she can name, although, when in charge of feeding a hyperactive young family, her appetite faded away as she put their needs before her own and, for the first time in her life, she became quite slim. Now she is older, food – particularly indulgent rich comfort food – is a great source of pleasure for her, and, as a result, she feels she has to be careful. She says of herself: 'I feel very fulfilled in the life that I have led, the only thing troubling me is my size.'

Physique

Earth-dominant types worry about their weight. Because they have a slow metabolism they tend to put on the pounds however carefully they eat. When they grow older they find it a real challenge to shed weight and may seem to be preoccupied in a constant battle against their own biology. They have large joints, heavy bone structures and female types are usually big-bosomed and round-hipped.

Other features

If you are Earth dominant you probably have large, liquid eyes with clear whites and heavy eyelids. Your veins and muscles are not particularly prominent and your body has a unique and recognizable scent that is more obvious than in the other types. Your skin tends to be thick and oily and your hair is lustrous, thick and strong. Your heart beat is steady, slow and regular, and you are perhaps more interested in cuddling and physical familiarity than in a wide exotic sexual repertoire.

Typical daily routine for Earth types:

Wake up: 90 minutes before sun rise.

Breakfast: Fresh fruit.

Teeth ritual: After you have brushed your teeth, massage your gums with ginger and rock salt.

Gargling: Gargle with ginger tea (steep half a teaspoon in a cup).

Morning drink: Warm herbal teas.

Bath/shower routine: Massage with a dry herbal powder like barley before bathing. Add a few drops of essential oil – lavender or sage – to your bath. Follow with an application of the massage oil recommended for your type.

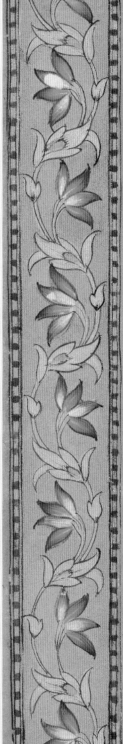

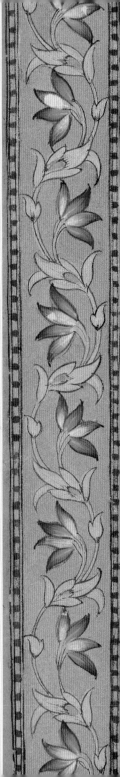

Face care: Follow cleansing, nourishing and moisturizing routine.

Meditation suggestions: Spend 20 minutes in meditation using the mantra recommended for your type.

Lunch: Choose from the Earth pacifying diet. Try to lie down for 15 minutes after eating with eyes closed.

Yoga practice: Fire breaths and the postures recommended for your type and some light aerobic exercise.

Dinner: Eat around 7.30–8.30pm choosing food appropriate to your type.

Sunset suggestions: Wash your body and put on loose clean clothes before spending 20 minutes in meditation.

Night time ritual: Follow cleansing, nourishing and moisturizing routine for your skin type. Earth types do not generally need massage to help sleep.

Sleep time: Try to turn your light out between 10–11pm.

Seasonal lifestyle recommendations for Earth types

During the spring and early summer, try to eat a diet that is lighter, less oily and drier than during the other seasons. Cut out excess heavy foods, such as yoghurt, ice cream, cream and cheese. Try to eat warm foods, especially those with a bitter and astringent tastes. Eat less sour, salty and sweet foods.

Typical health problems: eczema, sinusitis, hypertension, circulatory disorders, heart disease, diabetes, gall bladder problems, asthma, bronchitis, coughing, dyspepsia (poor digestion), excessive salivation.

Earth lifestyle checklist:

1. Try and go for a walk after you have eaten.
2. Make sure you undertake some physical activity each day, even if it is running up the stairs or ironing vigorously.
3. Stay in a warm environment and avoid cold, draughty rooms.

4. Try to avoid snacking between meals; if you are hungry eat some dried fruit rather than carbohydrates.
5. Eat as much spicy, hot foot as you like, but avoid fatty and fried food.
6. Take warm baths and wrap up warmly.
7. Get up early in the morning and try to avoid 'lie-ins' apart from as a treat.
8. Avoid eating too many Earth foods.

Earth case history 2

William, 40, is a property developer and antiques dealer. He believes that there is a right way of going about things, and enjoys tradition as well as creating new rituals in response to the new elements that emerge in his life. He is a sociable and gregarious soul, who retains anecdotes and details on the minutiae of other people's lives, but finds it hard to find an interest or memory for more abstract or illustrative information. He openly admits that he thrives on gossip. He enjoys the sensory side of life, fine wine, good food and takes considerable comfort in his environment. He is a natural and generous host. He always sleeps deeply and his girlfriend has to wear earplugs to cope with his frequent snoring. He is 6'2" tall and very well built, with thick curly hair, a broad chest and strong hairy limbs, but although he is strong his muscles are not particularly well-defined. He has large expressive eyes, slightly oily but smooth skin and is working to stay in shape as he is aware he has a natural disposition to putting on weight. He says of himself: 'I like the finer things in life and I enjoy working hard so that I deserve them.'

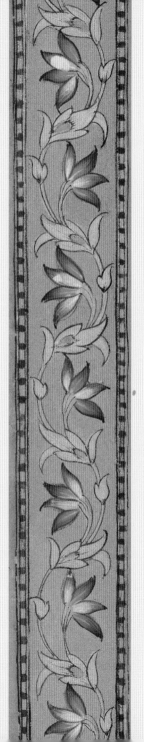

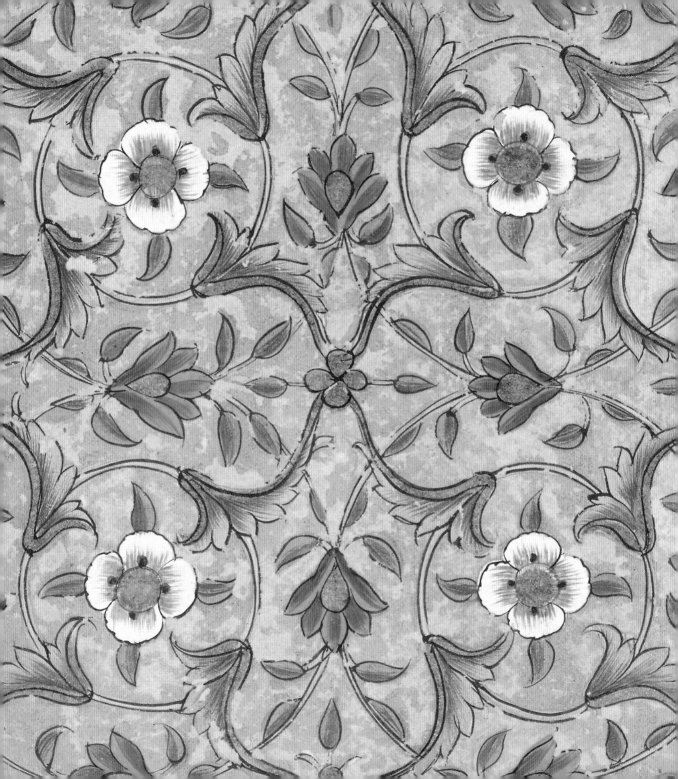

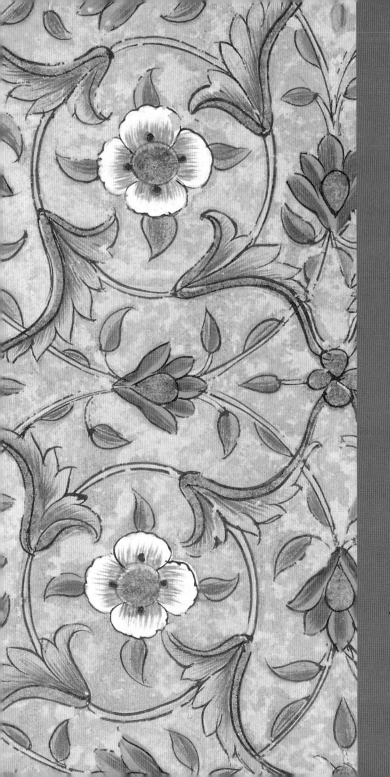

Ayurvedic Healing

Body, Mind and Soul

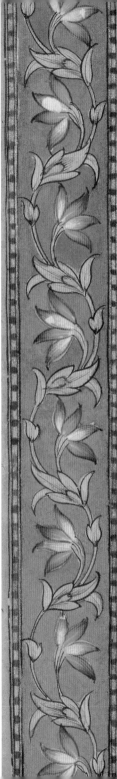

Beauty

All Ayurvedic health approaches and techniques will help make you naturally more radiant, but this chapter will focus more particularly upon perfecting the exterior with a skin care programme that works from the interior out, while revealing the inside story on dry, oily or problem skin, and what you can do about them. But do remember, there is so much more to beauty than external appearance. Later chapters will show ways in which to harness and develop the magical potency of your own inner radiance using Ayurvedic practices.

Ayurvedic practitioners have known the secret of beautiful, lustrous skin for more than three millennia, because they recognize that the skin is the reflection of everything that is going on inside us. The Ayurvedic approach to ageless beauty works because it is sensitive to individual needs, and always tailors the beauty routine to type. But when it comes to external skin care, the integrity of the Ayurvedic approach still applies: If you want energy, beauty and wellbeing you need to eat well and care for your own internal environment. However, this chapter will focus more particularly on the steps you can take to care for your visible outer shell. Used in combination with the rest of Ayurveda's holistic approach you will have, at your fingertips, a complete system to help prolong and maintain inner and outer radiance.

The key to Ayurvedic beauty treatments is helping the body to harness its own ability to balance and heal itself. If someone comes to my clinic with a

If you want energy, beauty and wellbeing

severe case of acne rosacea my immediate focus is not upon temporarily calming down the surface of the skin to improve its condition visibly, but understanding why that client's skin was particularly prone to become inflamed and what changes they can make to diet and lifestyle to stop their future susceptibility.

The Rishis, or sages, who originally formulated Ayurveda believed that your type (Air, Fire, Earth) determines your basic characteristics including your type of skin. They suggested that skin is the external evidence of the state of our inner being, a mirror by which others can read our soul. All our significant emotions and experiences are projected via our nerve endings and glands upon our largest organ, the skin: deep lines and wrinkles around the mouth and brow suggest someone who is often unhappy; a livid angry rash speaks of internal stresses; severe acne tells us of hormonal disorder; pallid sallow grey skin suggests a poor diet and someone who does not respect their body as it deserves. To the Ayurvedic health practitioner, skin problems are clear signals of imbalance deep within mind and body, far beyond the reach of the unguents with which we often try to soothe them away.

And so many of the potions we use are completely wrong in themselves, containing all manner of artificial additives and either washing away the very lubricants we would do well to retain, or clogging up our pores making it difficult for skin to breathe, in their mistaken approach to cleansing the skin. Shop-bought moisturizers and cleansers are rare in Ayurvedic households – those impossibly elegant, radiant Indian matriarchs have been mixing their own for years, sharing between them the secrets of the herbs and oils that they find naturally enhancing. I will show how you can do the same, applying only the purest, most vital extracts to your skin, working in harmony with it, not against it.

Glowing, healthy skin is the natural condition of all three types (Air, Earth, Fire) when mind, body and spirit are healthy, happy and fulfilled. When we are truly balanced our skin glows and is blemish-free, reflecting the peace and natural beauty that suffuses us, whatever our type. This is the goal! But the

Beauty basics:

The key to Ayurvedic beauty treatments is helping the body to harness its own ability to balance and heal itself.

you need to eat well and care for your internal environment.

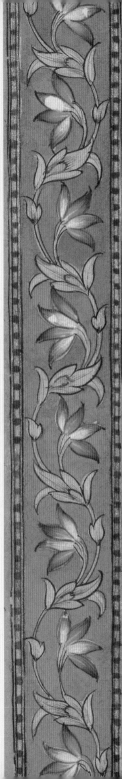

differences in the types mean that our skin responds differently to the reality of modern life; emotional and work pressures, environmental stresses, stimulants, artificial diet – all the elements that exacerbate the visible signs of ageing, wrinkles and skin disorders. When under pressure, the different skin types will react differently and display different sorts of problems.

Because of this, forget the idea that there is a single magical potion in a bottle that will suit everyone. Not everyone is born with the same type of skin. The first step to help reduce the signs of ageing and enhance your skin's luminosity is to know your Ayurvedic type – this is the key to creating better skin. If you are a mixed type, as most people are, your skin is likely to be your most dominant type. If, for example, you are an Air-Fire type, your skin is likely to be Air.

Air (vata) produces dry skin; Earth (kapha) produces oily skin; and Fire (pitta) produces sensitive or combination skin that is prone to inflammation or redness. In a well-balanced skin these effects will be superficial, for when your type is in balance all three skin types look clear: If you touch fiery skin it will simply feel a little warmer and more moist than the cooler and rougher airy skin, while earthy skin will be more waxy and lubricated than either Fire or Air. It is when your type is not balanced and you have an excess of dosha that the nature of the skin becomes more pronounced. If you have an excess of Air (vata) your natural dryness may lead to dermatitis, psoriasis or dry eczema. An excess of Earth (kapha) can lead to wet eczema, while too much Fire (pitta) can lead to burning rashes.

So once you know your type and where your balance lies, how do you maintain it? The answer is fundamental to the practice of Ayurveda. You should lower your intake of the elements that your body naturally has in abundance, and replenish the elements that your body lacks. If your skin is a dry Air skin, for example, and you race about, eating junk food, living by deadlines, drinking lots of tea and coffee you will soon overload an already excitable type with even more frenetic energy and your skin will become drier and drier. What you need is more Fire and Earth influences in your life.

We all have a certain amount of each type within us, but when it comes to our skin each of us has a dominant type. Answer the following four skin questions from the main type questionnaire to indicate your skin type, choosing in each case the answer that applies most:

A My skin is cool, rough and dry
B My skin is warm and prone to oiliness
C My skin is smooth, cool to the touch and not dry

A My underlying skin tone is best described as bluish
B My underlying skin tone is best described as reddish
C My underlying skin tone is best described as yellowish

A My skin is prone to dehydration and dryness, especially when it is cold outside
B I suffer rashes and inflammation and can burn easily
C I sometimes suffer whiteheads and blackheads

A My complexion is marked by fine lines, prominent veins
B I have some broken capillaries, freckles and moles
C My skin is supple and soft

Mainly As: Dry skin (Air)
Mainly Bs: Sensitive skin (Fire)
Mainly Cs: Oily skin (Earth)

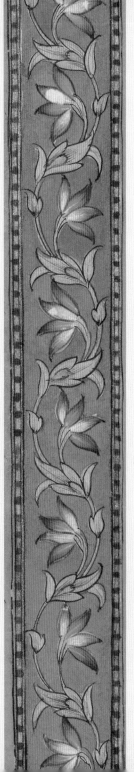

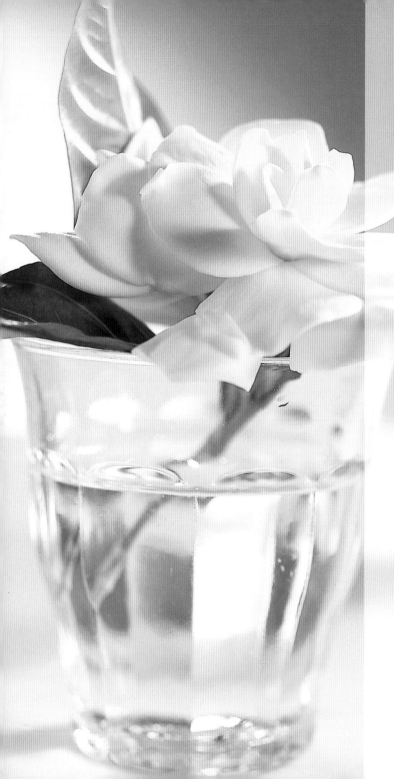

The Three-Step Guide to Healthier, More Lustrous Skin

Using an Ayurvedic skin-care routine to maintain a healthy and youthful complexion couldn't be more simple. There is nothing fancy or complex about it, just good common sense and the use of natural wholesome products. The three steps that apply whatever your skin type are cleanse, nourish and moisturize. This is the minimum required to alleviate the effects of stress, environment and the skin's own process of cell renewal. But remember, this process is purely external and will only help alleviate the symptoms of ageing and disease, and not tackle the underlying cause itself. Because Ayurveda is a holistic approach to health and wellbeing, it is therefore vital to cleanse and nourish and care for the body and mind internally. So alongside your sweet smelling home made oils, go that extra step and read my chapters on meditation, massage and breathing.

1. Cleansing

Too often, washing your face involves the use of harsh soaps that completely strip the natural oils from the skin and upset its balance as well as washing in water that is an inappropriate temperature for your body type. When you clean your face you are trying to remove any dead skin cells (skin sheds dead cells at the rate of one million per hour) and chemical toxins not sloughed off naturally by the skin, while also removing environmental debris – make-up, dirt and bacteria – that creates blocked, clogged pores.

Note well that if your skin is left squeaky clean you have robbed it of its natural lubricant, and it will respond by producing even more oil to compensate. Your pores will block up faster than before, and could trigger a skin complaint or exacerbate an existing one. So oily (Earth) skin doesn't benefit from harsh cleansing, neither does sensitive (Fire) skin thrive under the influence of harsh soap, nor does dry (Air) skin which is already suffering a lack of production of natural oil.

Before you wash, remove make-up and surface toxins by adding a few drops of the appropriate organic oil for your type to a cotton wool ball and wiping gently. Depending on your skin type choose the following vegetable oil:

Dry skin – Air types should use sesame oil.
Sensitive skin – Fire types should use sunflower oil.
Oily skin – Earth types should use corn or canola oil.

All types should then wash twice daily using natural sandalwood – or neem – soap which is gentle. Better still is the use of the right Ayurvedic herbal powder for your skin which will help gently scrub away without robbing the skin of its natural moisture content (see below).

Beauty basics:

When you clean your face you are trying to remove any dead skin cells and toxins not sloughed off naturally by the skin, while also removing make-up, dirt and bacteria that creates blocked, clogged pores.

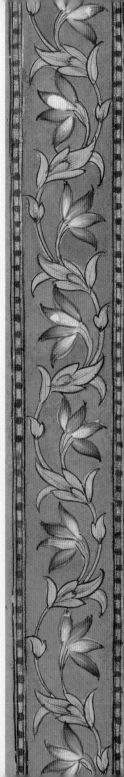

Dry skin – Air types should wash in hot water to improve circulation.

Sensitive skin – Fire types should wash in cool water so as not to over-excite circulation.

Oily skin – Earth types should wash in warm water to maintain circulation.

Herbal powder cleansing recipes:

Make up the recipe appropriate to your skin type and store in an empty film canister or spice jar. Twice a day use a large pinch of your bespoke cleanser mixed in the cup of your hand with warm water. Apply the paste over your face and neck and gently massage (do not scrub). Rinse well and leave to dry naturally.

Dry skin – (Air) Mix one teaspoon of finely ground almonds with a pinch of caster sugar and half a teaspoon of dry milk.

Sensitive skin – (Fire) Mix one teaspoon of finely ground almonds with half a teaspoon of dry milk and half a teaspoon of fresh orange peel. (Use only in the evening if your skin is super-sensitive, and wash using double dairy cream in the morning).

Oily skin – (Earth). Mix one teaspoon of finely ground barley meal with half a teaspoon of dry milk and one teaspoon of lemon peel.

2. Nourishing

After you have washed your skin, feed it with the best food on offer – pure and natural essential oils. Many shop-bought lotions consist of artificial ingredients that are actually too large on a molecular level to permeate the tissue, and instead they sit upon your skin like an oil slick, blocking your pores and acting like a trap to dirt and pollutants. Hopeless. Instead, essential oils are rich in nutrients and can travel through the skin to the deeper cells. When massaged into the skin, a second benefit is that the connective tissue is massaged and circulation stimulated, both of which help prevent wrinkles from forming. What's more, essential oils leave no oily residue on the skin's surface – within a minute they will have travelled deeper into the skin to do their real work. One of the best things you can do for your skin, whatever its type, is to nourish it with the right sort of oil. This applies even if your skin is already naturally oily.

Invest in bottles of essential oils which you can mix in ghee – clarified butter – which is available from health food stores or Indian supermarkets (it has an unlimited shelf life) or you can make your own. Alternatively, mix your chosen essential oil with the vegetable oil appropriate for your type (above).

Dry skin – (Air). The following oils are perfect for dry skin as they are soothing, sweet and warming: red sandalwood, neroli, vanilla, geranium, ginger, saffron, nutmeg and lemon.

Sensitive skin – (Fire). Choose from this list of oils which are soothing, cooling and sweet: sandalwood, ylang-ylang, mint, coriander, camphor, cumin.

Oily skin – (Earth). Oily skin benefits from oils that are warming, stimulating and fairly pungent: lavender, eucalyptus, bergamot, patchouli, clove, camphor.

The recipe:

To create your own face oil add 25 drops of essential oil to 25g of base oil (ghee or vegetable oil). Dab a few drops of face oil on your cupped hand, add a sprinkle of water and apply to moist skin. For body oil add 10 drops of essential oil into 25g of base oil and apply directly to moistened skin.

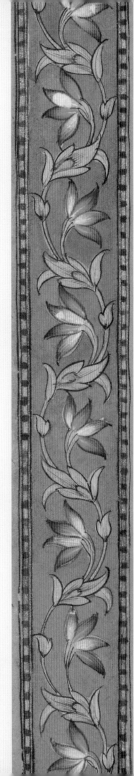

3. Moisturizing

When you nourish your skin with essential oil every day, you have actually moisturized your skin already. But you can protect your skin still further by gently massaging in a few drops of vegetable oil as well.

Dry skin – (Air) Use sesame oil.
Sensitive skin – (Fire) Use sunflower oil.
Oily skin – (Earth) Use corn oil or canola oil.

Extra Treats:

Weekly Fruit Mask

Once a week after you have followed the cleansing routine for your skin, mix up the following fruit pulp mask appropriate for your skin type. Apply generously to your face and neck, lie down for quarter of an hour to increase blood circulation to your face. Then wash with warm water before nourishing and moisturizing.

Dry skin: One banana or half an avocado blended to a pulp.
Sensitive skin: One banana or quarter of a pineapple crushed to a pulp.
For oily skin: Half a papaya or a handful of strawberries mashed to a pulp.

Monthly Fruit Peel

Once or twice a month use a natural fruit peel to give a deeper exfoliation – mix a few drops of freshly squeezed lemon mixed with a few drops of water swabbed onto the skin with cotton wool. But this is too strong for any skin to be used more frequently than that.

Beauty basics:

Ayurveda stresses the necessity for cleansing and nourishing and caring for the body and mind internally.

Gently massaging in a couple of drops of

Holistic Ageing Processes that Affect the Skin

External processes: The skin is the only organ of the body that is exposed to the elements, the destructive power of pollution, the sun, and the chemicals in our beauty products.

Internal processes: The amount of stress in your lifestyle has the power to alter the life cycle of your skin cells. Over time this builds up into a visible change in the outward appearance of your skin.

Solution: The facial skin demands and requires special attention, that the rest of the body does not, in order to help protect against premature ageing. You can't do much to control the weather, but the good news is that you can directly influence the youth and health of your skin with direct application of appropriate essential oils, what you eat, how you feel, your strategies for avoiding stress, and with positive affirmations through meditation.

Face Softening Mask

If your skin appears in need of a pep up, try this ancient and gentle solution. Mix a tablespoon of besan flour into a paste with natural yoghurt, turmeric powder and a dash of lemon juice. Apply to your face for 10 minutes and wash off in warm water. Your pores will be cleared of debris and your skin will feel wonderfully soft.

Beauty basics:

Natural fruit peels allow deeper exfoliation, but should not be used too frequently.

vegetable oil helps to protect and moisturize your face.

Why Stress is Your System's Greatest Enemy

Beauty basics:

Poor diet, lack of exercise, overwork, lack of sleep, over use of stimulants, unsatisfying relationships, personal crises and lack of purpose all go into a big internal melting pot of stress.

Beauty basics:

Stress is the fundamental cause of imbalance within our bodies and upon our external surface, our skin.

Let's imagine we are babies once again. We have been born with a perfectly balanced type. And whether we are Fire, Earth or Air, we are in harmony. Our skin is perfectly soft and unspoiled. It is blemish and problem free. Then we grow up, and as we do so our skin takes a battering as it is exposed to the unforgiving ravages of the environment and to our frenetic modern lifestyles. Gradually, over thirty years, it begins to deteriorate. Suddenly we have lines, we lose tone, our capillaries begin to break. What went wrong? Stress. Stress is the fundamental cause of imbalance within our bodies and upon our external surface, our skin. Stress – be it physical, spiritual or psychological – disturbs natural rhythms, according to Ayurveda. Poor diet and lack of exercise, overwork, lack of sleep, jet lag, shallow breathing, over-use of stimulants, environmental pollutants, unsatisfying relationships, food additives, personal crises, despair, doubt, confusion and lack of purpose all go into a big internal melting pot of stress known as '*santrasa*'. This is the continued discomfort of mind and body that upsets the body and disturbs the balance of our type. In Western scientific terms we call santrasa hormonal changes. Hormonal changes caused by stress are bad news for our skin.

When we are under stress, we start pumping out adrenaline and other hormones. As a result, our senses go on alert. We breathe faster and start digesting more slowly. Our blood sugar levels suddenly peak to provide more ready energy. Our heart pumps faster, so that the muscles are inflated for possible fight or flight. Our bodies are immediately suffused with the power to survive attack. But when we habitually live in a state of suspensive tension – because of deadlines or personal crises in our lives, racing to the catch the train, or worrying about losing our jobs – we continue to invest our bodies with

Secret Quick Cleanser

If you are short of time and require an extra radiance boost try this super quick cleansing technique. Pour boiling water into a basin over the juice of half a lemon and a splash of rosewater – add real rose petals if you have them to hand. Hold your face over the steam with a towel to trap the vapours, breathe deeply and pat dry afterwards. This is a wonderful cleanser which keeps your skin fresh and also invigorates you internally.

huge amounts of hormones and these begin to cause cellular breakdown. We are literally living faster than we are supposed to, without giving ourselves the space of a long-term break. It means that we age quicker because we are literally living in a state of potential emergency. Our immune system is fundamentally damaged by this state of hyper-arousal, when we are flooded with stress hormones we can't heal so well – and our skin ages quicker because in times of crisis our skin tissue is the last organ to receive nutrients. Instead, the blood supply to the other organs is increased, ready to fight or flight. That's why we go white as a sheet when we are scared. Extra blood flow leads to broken capillaries, and increased perspiration on the soles of our feet and under our arms can trigger eczema. It's not a pretty picture.

So what can Ayurveda, and its centuries of wisdom, teach us about our frenetic, carcinogenic modern lifestyles? In Ayurvedic terms, the process of disease and ageing begins when stress disturbs the balance of our natural type. It develops into full-blown physical disease when these imbalanced types disrupt

Beauty basics:

Stress – be it physical, spiritual or psychological – disturbs natural rhythms, according to Ayurveda.

the functioning of the seven body tissues (known in Ayurveda as the seven 'dhatus'). These are plasma, blood, muscle, fat, bone, bone marrow, nerve tissue, and reproductive tissue. When we are balanced, our type lives quite happily in a specific part of our body. Air (vata) lives in our colon and kidneys. Earth (kapha) in our lungs and stomach. Fire (pitta) in our liver and small intestines. But when we are under stress we build up excess Earth, Fire or Air in its natural home. If nothing is done to correct the imbalance aggravation occurs, and the Air, Fire or Earth elements start leaching out into the surrounding tissues. Eventually they take up new residence in tissue where they do not belong, but where bodily toxins caused by stress have created a weakness.

Beauty basics:

In Ayurvedic terms, the process of disease and ageing begins when stress disturbs the balance of our natural type.

Simply

58

Ayurveda

Hair Lustre Oil

Here is a wonderful potion that generations of Indian mothers have passed on to their daughters. It will make your hair incredibly soft and shiny.

Pour two teaspoonfuls of natural coconut oil into a saucepan, heat gently and add rosewater or a handful of real rose-petals. Then add a little massala spice powder, cover with a lid and simmer for three minutes. When cool, coat your hair in this beautifully fragrant concoction for an hour. Then shampoo and wash in the usual way. Your hair will have a wonderful lustre and scent.

The Secret of Bright Sparkling Eyes

A wonderful piece of Indian maternal wisdom is this simple trick for keeping your eyes white and bright. Simply apply cold milk to your eyelids with cotton wool each morning like a toner.

The chart below shows the way in which the different types are affected by large doses of stress.

Dry skin types (Air) become worried, fearful, distracted, insomniac and anxious under stress. The pituitary gland releases hormones that affect the kidneys.
Result: Excessive dehydration.
This shows as: Chapped lips, cracked feet, brittle nails, constipation, bloating, trembling, psoriasis, wrinkled skin, dandruff, split ends, gas, joint problems.
In extremis: Epilepsy, bloating, kidney problems.

Sensitive skin types (Fire) become frustrated, angry, critical and impatient under stress. Adrenaline is released.
Result: Flushed hot skin.
This shows as: Allergic reactions, acne rosacea, broken capillaries, burning eczema, white heads, rashes, heavy sweating.
In extremis: Liver disease, hypertension, inflammatory diseases.

Oily skin types (Earth) become lethargic, possessive, negative and depressed under stress. Excess production of sebaceous secretions.
Result: Water retention.
This shows as: Flabbiness, swollen feet and ankles, double chin, excess oiliness, acne, weight gain, bloating, colds, coughs.
In extremis: Diabetes, heart disease, urinary stones.

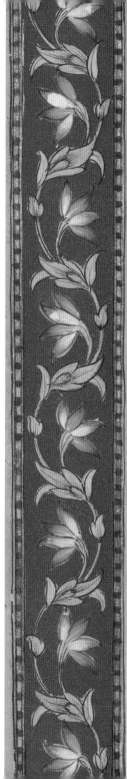

Ayurveda and Women

For all the increases in female emancipation, the fact still remains that the health of the family continues to revolve around the health of the mother. Women today have more opportunities than ever before, but also more stress and responsibility. We are under constant pressure to try and be superwoman; running a home, caring for and adoring our children, holding down demanding jobs and loving our husbands. All this against a backdrop of a time-poor, cash-rich society, where there is so much to do and so little time in which to do it all.

Traditional Ayurveda makes a distinction between men and women, women are viewed as the creators because they are the nurturers of life. A woman's health is seen clearly as her ability to keep her creative energies flowing. It calls upon a woman to look within herself for the key to her health. And Ayurveda is respectful of the natural cycles and rhythms of a woman's body: healthy menstruation regularizes a woman's emotional and physical ebbs and flows.

Ayurveda is the principle source of traditional medicine in India, Nepal and Sri Lanka. Many of the principles and many of its 'Vedic truths' have been handed down through the maternal line in the oral law of memorized hymns and poems for millennia. It offers a rich see-bank of knowledge for every stage of a woman's reproductive life. Follow my holistic advice for embracing, understanding and responding to the biological changes and demands of your femininity.

In traditional Ayurveda women are viewed

Menstrual Cycles

There are three types of premenstrual syndrome, but they can all be helped by taking regular exercise. However, you should try and rest and not over-strain yourself during the period itself.

Read the checklist below to assess what type, or mixture, of PMS you are suffering and how best to treat it. Please note that these function independently of your own type and you might experience them all at different times. But if you tend towards one particular type of symptom, you can start to help yourself by beginning to treat your body with the recommended cures a week ahead of the expected beginning of your period.

Airy PMS

Air influenced cycles tend to be more irregular than the other types, or regular cycles that occur with more time between them. Blood flow is often light and spotting is common just before the main flow as is constipation. More than any other type, it is Air women who are more likely to be so thin or to over-exercise to the extent that their periods cease for some time. Osteoporosis is most common amongst this type, particularly among young women, so Air types would do well to ensure they consume enough calcium, just in case.

Symptoms: Mood swings, lower abdominal pain, backache, distended rather than bloated tummy, anxiety, insomnia.

What to do: Swallow a tablespoon of aloe vera juice with a pinch of black pepper three times a day before you eat your meal. A handful of cherries before breakfast helps airy PMS as well as earthy PMS.

Herbal cure: Make up some dashamoola tea – just steep half a teaspoon of dashamoola in a cup of hot water and use honey to sweeten. Drink before breakfast and before retiring in the evening.

Basics for women:

Ayurveda is respectful of
the natural cycles and rhythms
of a woman's body: healthy
menstruation regularizes a
woman's emotional and
physical ebbs and flows.

as the creators because they are the nurturers of life.

Fiery PMS

Fire influenced cycles tend to be regular but occur more close together and produce heavy periods over many days. Fire women may experience loose stools just before their period begins and sometimes experience fairly strong cramps.

Symptoms: Breast tenderness, pain when urinating, hot flushes, irritability, food cravings, a burning feeling of excess heat in the body and mind, acne flare ups and headaches.

What to do: Each day, swallow a tablespoon of aloe vera juice with a pinch of cumin powder after breakfast.

Herbal cure: Mix two teaspoonfuls of shatavari with one teaspoonful of both brahmi and musta. Mix half a teaspoon of the concoction with half a glass of water each day.

Earthy PMS

Earth influenced cycles produce regular periods with dull pains and mild cramps and are more likely than the other cycle types to lead to yeast infections.

Symptoms: Water retention, enlarged, tender breasts, problematic drowsiness.

What to do: One tablespoon of aloe vera juice with a pinch of black pepper, pippali and ginger. You can also benefit from eating a handful of fresh organic cherries before breakfast each morning.

Herbal cure: Mix two teaspoonfuls of punarnava and two teaspoonfuls of musta with one of kutki. Mix half a teaspoon of the concoction with half a glass of water each day.

Nose Warming Cure for all PMS symptoms

All types of PMS can be smoothed along by dropping four drops of melted ghee into each nostril once a day and then breathing deeply to stimulate re-balancing of your system.

The Power of Guggulu

This Ayurvedic herb is very beneficial in helping to regulate menstruation and relieving some of the pain of PMS. Guggulu is available in several different formulations. Airy types should use triphala guggulu; Earthy types will benefit from punarnava guggulu; Fiery types can use kaishore guggulu. Take one tablet a day.

See also the advice on the two Ayurvedic herbs recommended as female aphrodisiacs, they are kumari and shatavari.

Some Indian women swear by the power of roast cumin seeds, just pop them in a dry pan over the heat until they begin to smell delicious (a great guide). Let them cool down and chew a small handful before washing them down with a tablespoon of aloe vera gel.

Sore breasts

You may be suffering PMS, hormonal imbalance or lymphatic congestion, or perhaps you are feeling sad or anxious. Sore breasts can incubate for a number of reasons. The good news is that there are two Ayurvedic self-treatment suggestions you can use for effective soothing. But first of all, take off that bra and if it seems tight treat yourself to a new cotton one that allows you room to breathe – literally.

Massage

Warm up two teaspoonfuls of castor oil and massage your tender tissue. Use gentle looping circles working from the breastbone out towards the arm, then guiding your fingers around the entire breast, including the nipple. This is also a good habit for checking for any changes in breast tissue as you get older

Herbal soothing

Sometimes tender breast tissue is the result of water retention. As the breasts engorge with excess fluid, the skin tightens and general discomfort

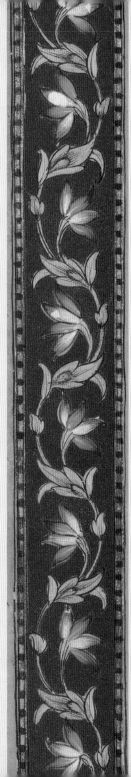

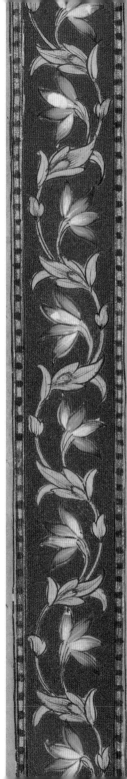

results. Try this recipe to alleviate the symptoms of water retention: Mix a third of a teaspoon of each of the following herbs – punarnava, shatavari, musta – and add half a teaspoon of the resulting mixture to a cup of hot water. You can drink this special breast brew twice a day.

Menopause

When the body stops producing female hormones in mid-life, we cease to release an egg each month and our periods stop. But the hormones that had controlled our monthly cycle had also controlled other biological elements, principally the metabolism of our bones. This is why you hear osteoporosis – brittle bone disease – bandied about in the same sentence as Hormone Replacement Therapy. When your supply of oestrogen dries up, so do your bones which become more porous and prone to breaking. Ayurveda explains it as a symptom of increased vata, that is as an Air-related condition. One of the benefits of synthetic HRT treatments is that they help prevent this process, and can even reverse it. I'm no great fan of HRT per se, but I do believe that it does have benefits in women likely to suffer from brittle bones. However, there are other more holistic and natural approaches that you should also consider – even if you decide to use these alongside any GP prescribed treatments.

In the West, the menopause is usually not treated until symptoms begin to arise with oestrogen's gradual withdrawal from the body. Only then are synthetic hormones prescribed. Ayurveda believes this is too late. In India, starting in their very early twenties, young women typically use herbal preparations to help normalize hormone levels throughout their entire lives. The monthly hormone fluctuations that can lead to PMS are smoothed, as is the transition into the menopause, with this approach. And it is true that Indian women who care for themselves in this way tend not to experience the abrupt hormone swings that can create the really severe menopausal symptoms.

The Ayurvedic Approach to Osteoporosis

Exercise helps keep bones strong, and this is also true for the menopausal woman. If you reward yourself with just 30 minutes of exercise, five days a week, you will be making a significant step to keeping your bones healthy and durable. Walking and swimming are perfectly sufficient, low impact exercise approaches. Exercising in a swimming pool, such as water aerobics, is also excellent as it encourages your bones to support loads without putting them under undue stress.

Calcium is a vital component in the formation of healthy bone – and should be combined with exercise. You can't do better than eat a calcium-rich diet in your mid-years after you've been out for that morning walk. Choose from milk, carrots, cheese, coconut, sesame seeds, soybeans and soy milk. Chewing a handful of white sesame seeds as you take your walk is particularly helpful – so many calcium rich foods are also dairy based and can lead to clogged arteries in the bid for healthy bones.

And why not try a regular glass of tasty almond milk: Soak 10 almonds overnight in water, peel them and blend with a cup of warm milk. Add a pinch of saffron, ginger, cardamom or cinnamon for a refreshing drink that is also kind to your bones.

You need approximately 1,200mg of calcium every day, and calcium supplements – natural ones are made from oyster shells – can be helpful if you find it difficult to consume sufficient calcium in your diet every day.

Herbal bone strengtheners

Phytoestrogens are plants that are rich in natural oestrogen, and Ayurveda has some recommendations here. An effective osteoporosis prevention technique is the following recipe. It sounds a bit complex, but you can mix up a batch once a week or so as you only need to take a quarter of a teaspoon twice a day.

Basics for women:

When your supply of oestrogen dries up, so do your bones which become more porous and prone to breaking.

Basics for women:

You need approximately 1,200mg of calcium every day in order to maintain healthy bones.

Mix five teaspoons of shatavari with three teaspoons of vidari and three of wild yam. Add half a teaspoon of shanka bhasma (conch shell ash) and kama dudha (coral shell ash). Measure out a quarter of a teaspoon each morning and night and add to a small glass of warm milk to maintain bones.

Dealing with symptoms of the menopause

Hot flushes, mood swings, water retention and insomnia: It's an unfortunate litany of the worst that the change of life has to offer. Try the following suggestions which have been tested by millennia of Indian women who did not have recourse to expensive, artificial drugs.

Diet

Because Ayurveda believes that symptoms of the menopause are connected to an excess of vata or Air energy, aim to eat a vata-pacifying diet. All types, not just Air types, will benefit from this (although it is particularly useful for Air types who tend to suffer more than most).

Aloe vera

You can bring a lot of relief to any menopausal problem by swallowing one teaspoonful of aloe vera juice three times a day.

Vaginal dryness

Try this ancient Indian technique for bringing relief: Take a piece of clean cotton and soak it in a few teaspoonfuls of sesame oil. Roll it up and tie a piece of cotton around one end. Insert inside your vagina at night.

Useful Yoga

Any of the yoga postures that concentrate on the lower abdominal area can offer some relief, but 12 cycles of the Sun Salutation each morning is particularly helpful (see chapter 8).

Basics for women:

Because Ayurveda believes that symptoms of the menopause are connected to an excess of vata or Air energy, aim to eat a vata-pacifying diet.

Mineral supplements

As well as taking extra calcium, you will benefit from topping up your diet with 600mg of magnesium and 60mg of zinc each evening. They help with hot flushes and help to prevent osteoporosis.

Hot flush cooler

Plagued by hot flushes? Try this remedy – keep the ingredients to hand so you can scoot down to the kitchen in the middle of the night if afflicted while you are trying to sleep: Mix one teaspoon of organic sugar into a cup of pomegranate juice and eight drops of lime juice. You can drink this up to three times a day and relief should soon follow.

Basics for women:

Regular exercise and a diet rich in calcium, magnesium and zinc help to reduce the symptoms of the menopause.

Vata Pacifying Diet

Avoid	Eat
Dried fruit	Sweet fresh fruit
Frozen, raw or dried vegetables	Cooked vegetables
Barley, cereals, couscous	Cooked oats, rice, pancakes
Corn, bread with yeast	Wheat, unleavened bread
Most pulses and nuts	Lentils, mung beans, soya, tofu
Powdered dairy goods	Most dairy is good
Yoghurt	
Lamb, pork, white turkey	Fresh meat and seafood
Chocolate	
Horseradish	
Caraway	All other spices are good
Maple syrup and refined white sugar	Raw honey, molasses, fructose

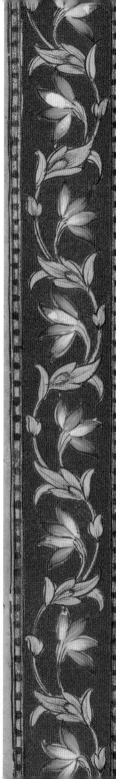

Supplements

More than 2000 different preparations are used in Ayurvedic medicine. Many include some of the most popular herbs in the world, such as aloe vera, turmeric, ginger and garlic. Other marvellously effective Ayurvedic supplements are far more exotic, and it is well worth trying the supplements mentioned below (see the resources chapter at the end of the book for more details on where to buy them). Although I have listed some of the herbs under dosha-type headings, these refer to imbalances that can be suffered by anyone (and are caused by an imbalance of that dosha) whatever their own constitution – so don't confine yourself to reading only about your type, think symptoms and see if there is something here that will help you.

Ayurvedic herbs are usually sold in combination formulas. I have avoided giving dosage instructions for the vast majority as it is preferable to follow the instructions on the packet.

Air Specific Natural Elements

This is an over-active dosha – the key is to calm the emotions and restore wellbeing. Spicy cinnamon, oriental ginger, exotic myrrh, sensuous rose, warm liquorice and mild vanilla are all useful.

Ayurvedic medicine uses some of the mos

Winter Cherry/Ashwagandha – The most famous Asian aphrodisiac is actually a warming root that has many benefits, including calming and relaxing Air types who can tend to overdo it. It clears the mind, encourages a restful night's sleep, and helps the stressed-out to unwind and restore energy. Said to be the Ayurvedic equivalent of ginseng.

Shatavari – A great source of natural vitamin A and an excellent rejuvenating tonic for women.

St John's Wort – A magical herb that is a great leveller in restoring calm to those prone to mood swings. Also said to be good for depression, anxiety and insomnia.

According to the Ayurvedic system of medicine, there are seven 'tissues' manufactured by the body: lymph, blood, bone, muscle, fat, nerve and reproductive tissues. A 30-day process transforms lymph into '*ojas*' – the body's most specialized tissue controlling reproduction, immunity and general health. Ashwangandha specifically builds ojas and therefore helps with these elements. In one study, it prevented stress-related gastric ulcers forming and the depletion of vitamin C. In another study, of 50-something men, greying hair and calcium levels were significantly improved. Seventy per cent of those using the herb also noticed increased libido and sexual function.

In Ayurvedic medical theory, Ashwandha balances both the nervous system (Air/Vata) and the musculoskeletal system (Earth/Kapha) while it also increases heat (Fire/Pitta).

It is common in chronic conditions for Air-Earth imbalances to be present. These are usually difficult to treat and end up being long-standing. A classic example is arthritis which involves joints which are both painful-dry (Air) and swollen-inflamed (Earth). Ashwagandha is a

Healing basics:

According to the Ayurvedic system of medicine, there are seven 'tissues' manufactured by the body.

popular herbs in the world and some of the most exotic.

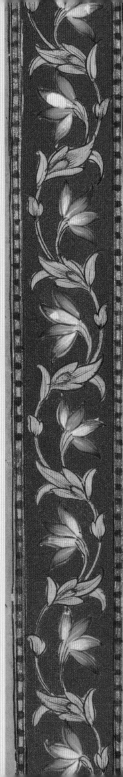

great medicine of choice as it balances both these problems.

It is also used effectively to treat insomnia but even this is with a twist – rather than tranquillizing you into sleep, instead it helps the body to settle and sleep, helping the body address a symptom of stress instead of masking the symptoms.

Ashwagandha

The wonder tonic that stops hair greying and improves your sex life.

A herb that rejuvenates the nervous system, erases insomnia and eases stress. Finding a gentle tonic for the ailments of the pressured 20th century, the ultimate elixir, sounds like a quest for the Holy Grail, but research has validated many virtues of the extraordinary Ayurvedic panacea, Ashwagandha. Sometimes known as Indian gingseng, in reference to its rejuvenative and tonic effects on the nervous system, in fact many scientific studies show it to be superior to its Chinese equivalent. It is believed to be helpful in the treatment of anti-inflammatory and digestive conditions, as well as nervous disorders, respiratory dysfunction and as a sedative and aphro-disiac. A small evergreen shrub, its potency lies in its roots which are most commonly used today. A typical dose is 250mg three times daily, but this depends upon the condition being treated.

Fire Specific Natural Elements

Intensity is the hallmark of Fire types – fiery by name, fiery by nature. They benefit from herbs and preparations that cool the emotions and restore serenity and harmony. Sharp peppermint, soothing sandalwood, pungent eucalyptus and cool ylang ylang are recommended for bringing peace and comfort.

Gotu Kola – Rumoured to be eaten in place of food by the Yogis, this meditative herb, when taken with honey, is said to be consciousness expanding. The leaves of this ultimate herb are believed to be helpful for all types, but are particularly good at soothing Fire-aggravated skin conditions.

Ginkgo Biloba – This is the tree of longevity, the plants themselves last a millennia and are rumoured to impart the secret of eternal life to humans. It is said to increase blood flow, boost oxygen levels in the brain and enhance circulation.

Bhringaraj – Ever watched the swishing radiant hair of Indian women and wondered why their locks are so lustrous? Bhringaraj is the secret weapon which every Indian mother knows will confer shiny healthy locks upon her daughters. Not only that, this is an excellent general tonic when taken internally and is soothing to the overwrought Fire types. It is also beneficial when applied to the skin as its antiseptic properties help to eliminate toxins.

Vetivert extract – This is a grass renowned for its ability to cool down hyped up Fire types. Its mild refreshing scent has been described, liltingly, as 'the smell of the first monsoon rains on parched soil'. Certainly it has a similarly soothing effect on the potentially snappish Fire types. It's also excellent when applied to the body in paste form as it can calm down inflammations. It is said to improve concentration and is traditionally sprayed on drapes and linen in Indian households, infusing entire houses with its fresh spring smell.

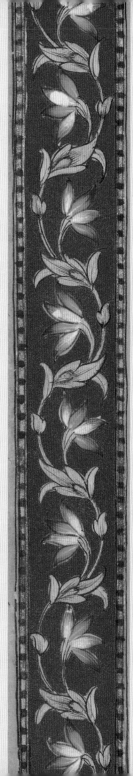

Earth Specific Natural Elements

Invigoration is the key for laid back Earth types who can tend to lethargy if not suffused with a sufficiently strong sense of adventure to create activity. Zesty lemon, stimulating basil, sensual amber, exotic cedar wood and passionate rose all help clear the way for mental clarity and encourage activity.

Guarana – This root has become well-known as a general caffeine substitute pick-me-up. It certainly gives instant energy, and boosts anyone feeling a little sluggish with a natural pep up.

Gingseng – A famous Chinese tonic that has been proven to increase resistance to stress. It is revitalizing, aids mental performance and memory, and restores energy. It is also believed to slow down the ageing process.

Boswellin – This is an ancient Ayurvedic remedy which has recently been picked up by the medical community because of its extraordinary properties in the treatment of arthritis – both rheumatoid and osteoarthritis. The conventional non-steroid approach to treating this highly uncomfortable deterioration of joint cartilege can have some unpleasant side effects. This old remedy appears to have marked success in reducing the pain of the conditions without the problems, and throughout history its extracts have provided relief from arthritis and other conditions leading to joint pain, such as gout. The tree from which the resin is taken grows widely in dry hilly areas in India and in ancient times it was literally worth its weight in gold. In a recent study 14 per cent of patients rated its effects as excellent, 53 per cent as good, 30 per cent as fair and only three per cent as poor. It took between two and four weeks for the pain of symptoms to begin to abate.

Healing basics:

Guarana gives instant energy, and boosts anyone feeling a little sluggish.

Other Persuasive Ayurvedic Tonics

Triphala is the most widely used herbal preparation in Ayurvedic medicine. It is known as as 'a good manager of the house' because it helps to harmonize different bodily functions. In particular it helps to enhance nutrient absorption, regulate metabolism and iron out any hiccups in digestion.

Neem is one of the Ayurvedic greats known in India as 'the village pharmacy' in deference to its versatility. It's been around for 4,500 years and it is as popular today as ever. It is used primarily in the treatment of skin diseases, fever and inflammation, and has applications as wide ranging as mouthwash, insect repellent and skin cream. In India it is particularly popular for treating acne and eczema and is good for Fire types who are suffering Fire imbalance leading to dry, itchy skin. What's more, scientific research in the West confirms that this is indeed a powerful, but safe, treatment.

Mangista is a crushed seed from a tree which grows widely in India. It is particularly good for skin problems but can only be prescribed in this country by an Ayurvedic doctor. If you have a bad case of eczema or psoriasis consider making an appointment with one of the medical clinics mentioned in the resources section.

Turmeric, a herb of the ginger family, and the major ingredient of curry powder, is grown all over India. It is used in both the Chinese and Indian systems of medicine as an anti-inflammatory agent and in the treatment of numerous conditions, including flatulence, jaundice, menstrual difficulties, toothache, bruises, chest pain and colic. It is particularly effective at lowering cholesterol levels. It is also a valuable herbal treatment in the war against cancer; several studies suggest that as well as inhibiting the development of cancer it can also promote cancer regression.

Details on where to buy these herbs are to be found in the resources section at the back of this book.

Healing basics:

Triphala is the most widely used herbal preparation in Ayurvedic medicine. It helps to harmonize different bodily functions.

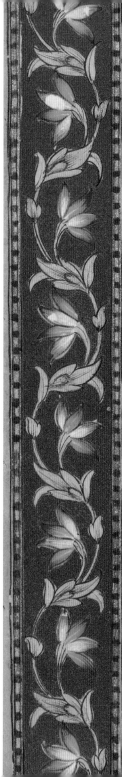

A-Z of Common Ailments

Because Ayurveda is such an integrated and holistic philosophy, your wellbeing, health and beauty can only be enhanced if you act swiftly to treat common ailments – the fluctuations in your constitution that show your internal balance is in need of a little tweaking and fine tuning. View this next section as your kitchen cupboard medicine cabinet, a collection of simple health cures you can make at home. Some of the herbs and ingredients may be unfamiliar to you, many you can find in a large supermarket, the rest can be sourced through Indian greengrocers. These are well worth a visit for the exotic and intriguing looking Asian fruit, vegetables and herbs they offer, many of which have medicinal properties.

 Acne Rosacea (excess Fire): This red inflammation of the skin appears as a sensitive rash on the nose and cheeks, and is often accompanied by excessive oiliness and broken capillaries. This is sensitive skin at its worst and you need to treat it carefully. So avoid any harsh substances, this skin wants only gentle, soothing care. To calm the skin, steep $1/3$ of a teaspoon of cumin, coriander and fennel in a cup of hot water for 10 minutes, strain and drink after each meal. You can make a healing face mask by mixing almond powder (grind almonds in a blender) with a few teaspoons of water, apply to your face and let dry for half an hour before rinsing.

Your health and beauty can only be

Anxiety attacks (overstimulated Air): Take a hot bath adding two heaped tablespoons of ginger and the same amount of baking soda to the water. Shut your eyes and breathe in the vapours for a quarter of an hour. If you are on the move and can't bathe, a quick fix to soothe a racing heart beat is a cup of orange juice with a pinch of ground nutmeg and a teaspoon of honey. If there is no ginger or orange juice available, lie on your back with your hands by your side, close your eyes and breathe deeply for a few minutes to regain your composure.

 Athlete's foot (overstimulated Earth and Fire types who perspire a lot): Swab the affected area with tea tree oil, a natural antiseptic. Then mix one teaspoon of aloe vera gel with a large pinch of turmeric and apply to the itchy parts of your feet before you go to bed. Use this approach for two weeks. Warning: you need to sacrifice a pair of socks, as this is a bright yellow mixture which will stain both your feet and your bed-clothes. Cool burning feet with sandalwood oil or mango juice.

 Bad breath (a symptom of weak digestion or 'reduced gastric fire' associated with excess Air): Avoid heavy meals and cold drinks, cheese, yoghurt and ice-cream – all of which reduce the gastric Fire. A natural remedy is to chew a mouthful of roasted fennel and cumin seeds after each meal. This will improve digestion and help to detoxify the colon. You could also chew cardamom seeds throughout the day, and twice a day drink half a cup of aloe vera juice until sweetness is restored to your breath.

Bee and wasp stings (which trigger a local irritation of Fire under the skin): A staple of the Asian diet is ghee or clarified butter which you rub on to the area that has been stung. Butter is a good substitute and helps reduce the sensation of stinging.

Blackheads: These irritating blocked pores are caused by excessive oil secretions (and are therefore symptomatic of excess Earth or kapha).

Healing basics:

Common ailments are the fluctuations in your constitution that show your internal balance is in need of a little tweaking and fine tuning.

enhanced if you act swiftly to treat common ailments.

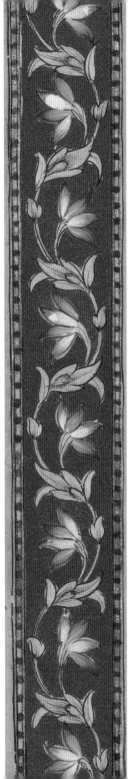

In dealing with them you need to take care not to damage the capillaries that feed them, so instead of squeezing them try these two home remedies: Add half a teaspoon of Epsom salts to a cup of warm water, wash your face by dipping a cotton ball in the liquid. Grind up fresh parsley into a pulp and apply to the oily area prone to blackheads, lie down for 15 minutes to encourage blood circulation to the face, then cleanse, nourish and moisturize as normal.

Cellulite (imbalance of Earth or Air): Drink half a cup of aloe vera juice in the morning to detoxify, massage your stomach and thighs with warming oils such as rosemary and bergamot, exercise more and avoid eating foods that inflame kapha.

Colds and flu (imbalance of Air and Earth in which the body builds up excess Earth which quells the digestion): Brown half a cup of coriander seeds in a frying pan, but do not let them roast. Then boil them in a pint of water with four slices of root ginger (the best remedy for colds) until the water has reduced by half. Use a sieve to strain the liquid, add sugar to taste, and drink.

Cold sores: Apply aloe vera gel to the blisters or, if you are feeling adventurous, ask your local Indian supermarket for bitter ghee and use it like an ointment several times a day.

Constipation (imbalance of excess Air leading to dryness and hardness): For constipated babies, apply a few drops of castor oil to the nipple which the baby will suckle along with the mother's milk. Adults should only add two teaspoonfuls of castor oil to a glass of hot water if they are quite severely constipated. For more general blockages, drink plenty of water and snack on fruit; the most effective fruit is ripe bananas, which have a mild laxative effect; apples, peeled and eaten about an hour after a meal, pineapple juice; prunes and peaches. And try to eat more fibre. If your constipation is quite severe, mix two teaspoonfuls of ghee into a cup of hot milk and drink at bed time – but avoid this if you are an Earth (kapha) type.

- **Coughing** (imbalance of excess Fire or Earth in the bronchial tree leading to irritation and congestion): For a dry cough eat a ripe banana covered in a drizzle of honey to lubricate the throat, add a few twists of ground black pepper to encourage salivation.
- **Chest pain:** Pour two cups of water into a saucepan, bring to the boil and add three or four cloves of garlic, boiling until soft. Then crush the cloves into the water and drink the reduced solution. It won't make you popular, but it is an effective treatment!
- **Cystitis:** Follow the coriander seed recipe for colds and flu, but drink this solution every day for a week. Your urine will soon become clear and alkaline, and the burning sensation will stop.
- **Dandruff** (imbalance of Air): You need to get the circulation in the scalp going again, so massage your head with a teaspoon of neem oil (available from Indian supermarkets) in a base of sesame oil – the antiseptic properties of the neem oil will also help reduce any fungal infection. Another alternative is mixing one egg yolk with a squirt of lime-juice and a few drops of camphor and applying to your scalp for ten minutes to help reintroduce missing protein to your scalp. Rinse with warm water.
- **Diabetes** – mild, non-insulin dependent only (an imbalance of Earth which leads to diminished digestive Fire): The karella is a bitter melon fruit which you can buy in Indian greengrocers and is renowned for its calming properties. Cut the karella into chunks and boil the flesh and seeds in water. Eat while warm twice a day.
- **Diarrhoea** (imbalance of Air leading to reduced digestive Fire): This can be gradually stopped using the following kitchen cupboard recipe: Pour a pint of water into a saucepan and add one tablespoon of cumin seeds, six dried curry leaves, a pinch of salt, one teaspoon of black pepper and two crushed cloves of garlic. Boil until the mixture reduces by half and drink. Use this recipe three times a day. Another remedy is to

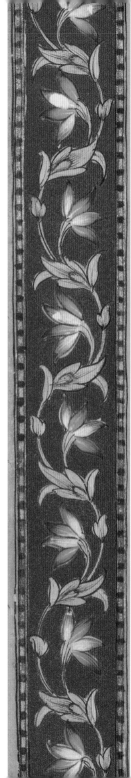

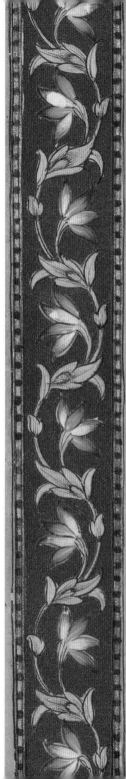

cook two apples until soft, add a teaspoon of ghee (or butter), a pinch of nutmeg and a pinch of cardamom (bananas make a good substitute).

Dizziness (imbalance of Air and Fire): A simple home remedy is mixing soda water with the juice of a lemon and sipping from time to time until the sensation of dizziness disappears.

Dry skin (usually an imbalance of excess air or Fire drying the body out): Do not spend money on expensive moisturizers. A better solution is to use oils found in the supermarket for a quick fix cure. Air types should use sesame; Fire types should use coconut; Earth types should use corn oil. But remember that dry skin is more likely to come from internal rather than external causes – to treat the cause of the problem, rather than the result, use an oil enema (see page 116 on Panchakarma). All types can give their skin an occasional treat using a mask of pulped cherries, applied and left for 15 minutes before going to bed.

Fever (a sign of toxins in the circulatory system): Ayurveda might have invented the mantra 'feed a cold and starve a fever' for that is the advice it offers. Fast while feverish, sip water or fruit juice but avoid milk as this can create diarrhoea and exacerbate the fever. Heat half a cup of mustard oil in a saucepan, soak a flannel in the solution and apply to the forehead, redipping the cloth when necessary to keep it moist.

Furry tongue: Ginger is a good anti-fungal agent. Just rub the tongue with a small, freshly sliced piece of ginger. This also works for general fungal infections in the mouth.

Gas and flatulence (whenever we eat anything we swallow a small amount of Air which increases vata – especially if our diet includes a lot of Air-aggravating foods, and all food we eat is gently fermented which also produces gas): To calm disturbances in the colon, grate some fresh ginger root, add a squirt of lime juice and swallow the mixture after eating. An even simpler remedy is to stir a pinch of baking soda and a teaspoon of lemon juice into a cup of cool water and swallow after meals. This mixture forms carbon dioxide which helps digestion.

Hangover (a fuzzy head and an inability to concentrate after consuming alcohol are symptoms of excess Fire): A glass of coconut water is a particularly effective rehydration tool. You could also try a glass of freshly squeezed orange juice with a pinch of cumin powder and a teaspoon of lime juice. Or add a teaspoon of sugar, a pinch of salt and half a teaspoon of baking soda to a glass of water just before drinking. Drinking diluted live yoghurt with a pinch of cumin powder throughout the day will rehydrate you and help you feel less drowsy and nauseous.

Headaches: A quick and easy solution is to follow the same remedy as for fever. But there are different types of headaches which the following remedies can help soothe.

Throbbing headache – If your headache is in the back of the head, throbs, and is accompanied by aching shoulders and a stiff neck you are probably suffering an **Air** type headache which can be caused by poor posture or dehydration: Mix half a teaspoon of lime juice, a tablespoon of sugar and quarter of a teaspoon of salt into a pint of water. If you are a vata type who suffers frequently from headaches it would be a good idea to follow a vata-reducing diet.

Penetrating headache – If your headache begins in the temples, moves behind the eyes and is penetrating or burning, you are likely to have a **Fire** type headache. Avoid sunlight, high temperatures and spicy food. A simple and effective remedy is to swallow two tablespoons of aloe vera juice two or three times a day. A bar of chocolate can also help by raising your blood sugar level. Alternatively, make a fiery headache tea by steeping half a teaspoon of coriander and the same amount of cumin in a cup of hot water.

Dull headache – A dull, deep-seated headache that feels worse when you bend over is likely to be an **Earth** headache, and may be associated

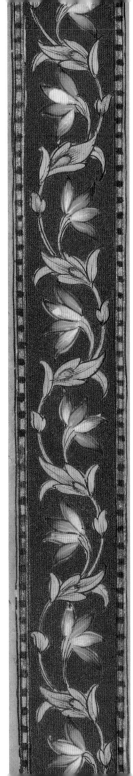

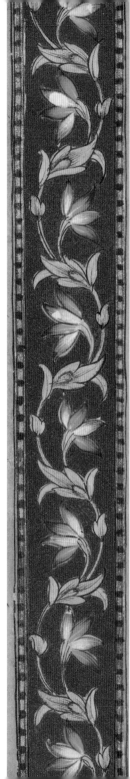

with sinus troubles. An unusual remedy which can be effective is to make a thick paste using half a teaspoon of salt and a teaspoon of water, and place a drop in both nostrils for 10 minutes. This helps to unblock the sinuses. Another way to relieve congestion is to pour a teaspoon of eucalyptus oil into a saucepan of boiling water, cover your head with a towel and inhale deeply. You can also add ginger, either fresh or powdered, to the mixture.

Heartburn (imbalance of Fire): Papaya juice is a particularly good way of controlling excess acidity. Mix it with two pinches of cardamom and sugar to taste. AVOID if you are pregnant, as papayas contain natural oestrogen. A remedy that is safe for everyone is to make your own effervescent powder (much cheaper than shop-bought solutions), add half a teaspoon of lime juice and the same amount of sugar to a cup of water, then add quarter of a teaspoon of baking soda and drink quickly while the drink is fizzing wildly.

High cholesterol: Try to eat as much garlic in your diet as possible, as garlic has been shown to reduce cholesterol levels – and avoid eating fat where possible.

Indigestion (excess Air leading to a reduction in the digestive Fire): Ginger is the answer here as it rekindles your digestive Fire. Buy it fresh and crush a small piece to extract the juice, before mixing with half a tablespoon of lemon juice and a pinch of salt. True ginger devotees may simply like the excuse to chew a small chunk of ginger, swallowing the juices that are released and spitting out the pith. Another approach is to pop a bay leaf in a cup of hot water and steep for 10 minutes before adding a pinch of cumin and drinking. For acute indigestion add the juice of a quarter of a lime to a cup of warm water and stir in half a teaspoon of baking soda before swallowing.

Insomnia: Often caused by the stresses of the modern age, Ayurvedic sages explain it as a build up of excess vata or Air dosha. The easy solution is a cup of warm milk, but this is made even more efficacious if you add some crushed almonds and a pinch of nutmeg. If you happen to have cherries in the fruit bowl, snack on them. Some Ayurvedic doctors prescribe drinking a glass of tomato juice with two teaspoons of nutmeg before eating your evening meal.

Period pains: Mix quarter of a cup of cumin seeds and one cup of dried curry leaves with a small saucepan of water. Boil until it reduces by half and swallow the mixture, sweetened with honey if necessary, several times a day.

Poor circulation: If your hands and feet often seem to be cold, a good trick is to massage them with a mixture of sesame seed oil and mustard seed oil warmed until they are hot. But do be careful not to burn yourself.

Psoriasis (imbalance of Air and Fire): These silvery flakes tend to appear in the hair-line, but in extreme cases can affect other parts of the body such as the eyebrows, they are caused by chronic dryness. After bathing apply ghee to the affected area, and take daily supplements of primrose oil, vitamin E and cod-liver oil which encourage the skin to lubricate.

Puffy eyes (excess Earth): Gently press underneath the eye, from inside corner to outside corner, to encourage the lymphatic fluids that are collecting here. Soak black tea bags in warm water (or, if you prefer, cotton puffs dipped in witch hazel) and placed them upon your closed eyes for 15 minutes.

Rheumatism: Use pure mustard oil as a massage oil, applying it to areas of the body that are affected once a day.

Sinus problems: Boil half a cup of coriander seeds in water, pour into a bowl, cover your head with a towel, lean over the bowl and inhale the steam.

Sore feet: Add half a cup of mustard seeds to a washing up bowl of hot water and immerse your feet for a reinvigorating soak until the water becomes lukewarm.

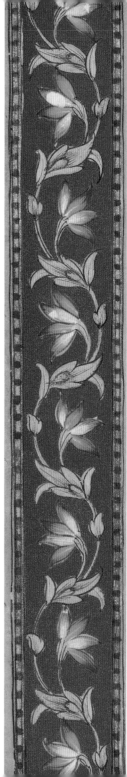

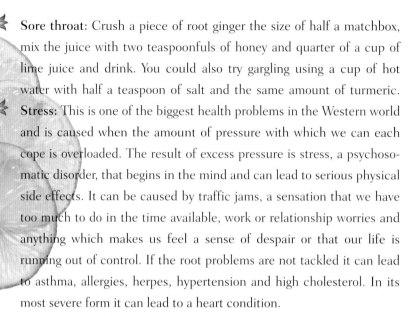

Sore throat: Crush a piece of root ginger the size of half a matchbox, mix the juice with two teaspoonfuls of honey and quarter of a cup of lime juice and drink. You could also try gargling using a cup of hot water with half a teaspoon of salt and the same amount of turmeric.

Stress: This is one of the biggest health problems in the Western world and is caused when the amount of pressure with which we can each cope is overloaded. The result of excess pressure is stress, a psychosomatic disorder, that begins in the mind and can lead to serious physical side effects. It can be caused by traffic jams, a sensation that we have too much to do in the time available, work or relationship worries and anything which makes us feel a sense of despair or that our life is running out of control. If the root problems are not tackled it can lead to asthma, allergies, herpes, hypertension and high cholesterol. In its most severe form it can lead to a heart condition.

There are different types of stress depending on your type:

Air stress – this tends to show itself as a form of anxiety, perhaps as a phobia or in the form of a panic attack.

Fire stress – this leads to a lack of control and anger which can also show itself in disorders such as ulcers and hypertension.

Earth stress – leads to a desire to eat away the pain, as well as to a slowed metabolism, underactive thyroid function and increased blood sugar.

Breathing stress cure: When you feel stress building up, sit back, switch off and take long deep breaths to prevent your body reacting physically. Think about a soothing scene that relaxes you and follow the breathing and meditation cures (pages 95 to 103).

If you can, have a bath (add one tablespoon of baking soda and the same amount of ground ginger to hot water) and afterwards rub vegetable oil (Earth = corn oil; Air = sesame oil; Fire = sunflower oil) into your body.

Analyze your stress. Make a list of all the elements that are creating stress in your life and separate them into two columns – stress you can do something about, stress you cannot change. Take control of what you can, and visualize yourself letting go and accepting the things you can't. Take care to note which form of stress might be being created by your imagination – negative thinking is a highly erosive force.

Make an anti-stress tea by steeping a teaspoon each of camomile, angelica and comfrey in a pot.

Crying is a good way of washing away your stress – if you feel close to tears let them come – and then encourage yourself to laugh. Even if it feels forced initially it has quite surprisingly relaxing powers.

Sunburn: Gently rub aloe vera juice into the sensitive area. Or dip a cotton pad into cold milk and apply it to the sunburn. Some practitioners believe that a pulped lettuce pack applied to the area is particularly helpful.

Toothache (aggravation of Air in the skeletal system): Dip a tiny piece of cotton wool into cinnamon or clove oil and wedge it into the space between gum and painful tooth. Another treatment is to take a clove of fresh garlic, crush it with the end of a wooden handled spoon and apply half the pulp to the tooth in the same manner.

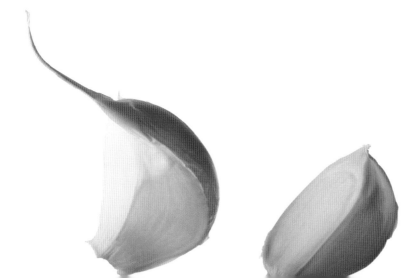

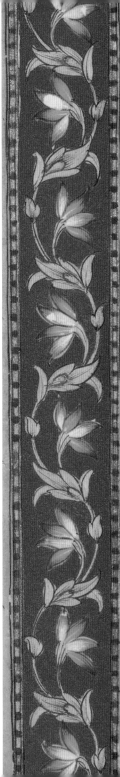

Yoga, Meditation and Breathing

Regarding your body as a temple, a place of respect, elevates your experience of life. Who feels good if they regularly slob in front of the television, eating plates of junk food and doing little more than reaching for the remote control? How much better we all feel if we stretch our legs, breathe in some fresh air, read a good book and ingest interesting healthy food. We need to care for our bodies. They are the machines that propel us through life, and like cars and bicycles they need regular maintenance. Ayurveda sees the mind, body and spirit as an interconnected whole. Changes in one element affect the others – both positively and negatively.

Ayurveda promotes the idea that everyone should do some exercise every day. All types should practise yoga. In addition **Earth** types benefit from aerobic activity, such as jogging, cycling or tennis; **Fire** types benefit from the cooling effect of swimming; and **Air** types can supplement their yoga exercises with walking. You know you've exercised sufficiently when you have light perspiration on your forehead and along your back. Pushing yourself regularly beyond this is not recommended.

In traditional Ayurvedic teaching there are a number of core elements used to give quality to our physical and psychological experience of life. The

Yoga is considered to harmonize the body,

great news is that yoga, breathing exercises and meditation are non-strenuous and the benefits of spending a few minutes each day practising them are immense. You can enjoy them individually, or you can follow my daily sequence, detailed below with variations, where appropriate, for differences in type.

Yoga

Yoga is already well known in the West as a form of exercise that is designed to bring the body and mind into harmony. It was developed more than two millennia ago as an aid to spiritual enlightenment and is still considered the most effective form of exercise within Ayurveda. Yoga is a way of bringing into harmony the body, mind and emotions in a simple, gentle, yet focused way that improves posture and increases suppleness.

Having viewed it sceptically, as it did the meridians and energy points in acupuncture, Western science is now finding that the seven invisible energy centres (or *chakras*) stimulated by yoga seem to correspond to the pathways of the immune system and the brain. There are two key elements of yoga – postures (known as *asanas*) and breathing exercises (known as pranayama). If you experience any pain while trying the following exercises stop and arrange to check with your GP if it is safe for you to practise yoga.

According to ancient teaching, yoga helps a form of spiritual energy (known as 'kundalini') to rise from the base of the spine to the top of the head. Countless people speak of the sensation of an 'energy surge' moving up their spine when they are in deep meditation or enjoying focused yoga practice. Along with this comes a feeling of contentment and calm. Practising yoga and meditation regularly is said to ensure that these energy centres are left clear and unblocked, in a form of invisible preventative medicine.

Exercise basics:

Yoga was developed more than two millennia ago as an aid to spiritual enlightenment and is still considered the most effective form of exercise within Ayurveda.

mind and emotions in a gentle yet focused way.

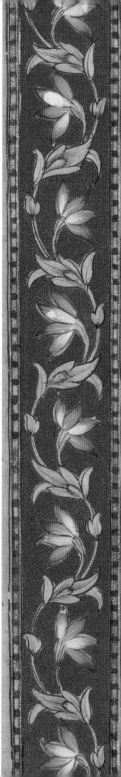

The Chakras

Imagine a rope running up inside the centre of your body. Upon it are seven knots which correspond to the seven energy centres or 'chakras'. These are the symbolic representation of the body's endocrine glands, or hormonal centres, and are sometimes known as 'energy wheels'. Everyone can experience the sensations related to the chakras without being aware of their origin. When you feel the sensation of butterflies in your stomach before a significant event, or become aware of a knot in your throat when you feel emotional but can't express yourself, or feel that delicious melting sensation of sexual arousal in your lower body, you are literally sensing the effect of your chakras. When you are waiting for the person you love at an airport and finally see them emerge, the physical feeling of warmth in your chest is your heart chakra reflecting the love that resides inside you.

The chakras do not stand alone. Like knots on that piece of string they are connected to one another. The secret of yoga is the belief that its correct practice will stimulate each chakra in turn and help to give us physical and emotional unity by sending our energy flowing upwards through each energy centre in turn, leading to a sense of spiritual tranquility.

Each chakra is known by a different colour – the colour that symbolizes its function. Becoming aware of your chakras and concentrating on each one in turn for a few minutes will help give you a reading about the state of your emotional and physical health:

The *red* chakra is the sexual centre. It is located in the genitals and is associated with life and survival. When energy flows through it you feel infused with passionate direction, aliveness, alertness and sexual desire.

Chakras are the symbolic representation

When the energy is blocked you can feel guilt about sex, emotionally needy and directionless.

The *orange* chakra is the lower body chakra, located just below the navel, and is the body's centre of balance and movement. Strength, vitality and physical grace flow through this chakra. But if the energy becomes blocked here you can feel hypercritical, stiff, tense and aggressive.

The *yellow* chakra is the solar plexus chakra, located in the hollow just below the rib cage. This is the centre of our self-esteem. Charisma, radiance, cheerfulness, self-confidence, and a sense of possibility and new horizons are experiences that flow from here. When blocked we feel nervous, timid and unconfident.

The *green* chakra is the heart chakra, located in the centre of the chest. When energy flows here sparks really fly, we feel love, joy, playfulness and laughter coupled with trust, compassion and empathy. But close this chakra up and we are left with great negativity, doubt, cynicism and bitterness.

The *violet* chakra, located in the throat, is our centre of self-determination and personal authenticity. We can give voice to our needs and desires when energy flows through here, we stand up for what we believe in, we demonstrate integrity in our feeling – even if that involves appearing anti-social or obstinate. Take away the energy from this centre and we are left directionless, we become listless, worthless and constantly put our partner's needs above our own. We feel that life is only skin deep and cannot touch us more deeply.

The *blue* chakra is located in the forehead, between and behind the eyebrows. This is the third eye, that part of ourselves that makes us feel free, creative, imaginative and intuitive - having insight without needing to use logic and reason. Block this centre and life seems dull and listless, devoid of meaning or higher purpose or personal fulfillment.

The *white* chakra is known as the crown chakra and is located on top of the head. This is the most magical of all the chakras. When the energy flows

of the body's seven energy centres.

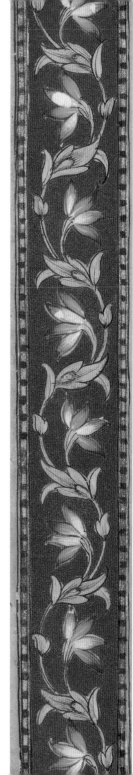

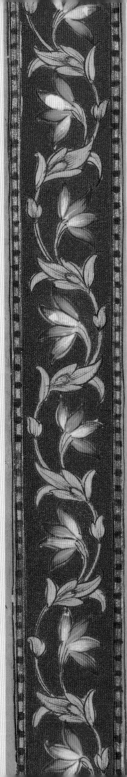

here we feel sensations of complete fulfillment and pure joy, it creates a delicious connection to everyone and everything in which we are at our best, most spontaneous and evolved selves. We feel invincible, capable of achieving whatever goals we set ourselves. But close this centre and you are exiled to an insubstantial fantasy world, grasping at the beauty that lies beyond the screen, unable to feel spiritually authentic or truly connected to yourself or your partner.

Always practise yoga on the floor as you need good support, remove jewellery and wear loose clothing. The best time to practise yoga is after you wake up and before breakfast.

Yoga stretching is recommended for all types, but certain postures are particularly beneficial for different types. Don't worry how you look when performing the postures, the benefits come from the gentle stretching and from tuning in to your body – 'becoming mindful' or 'in the moment.'

Everyone should start with the sun salutation, and at the very least your yoga practice should consist of twelve repeated cycles (at different speeds depending on your type – see below) of this fluid all-body exercise. In addition, to create a simple yoga regime, add at least the two additional postures for your type. Alternatively, if you are feeling energetic, you can work through the entire set.

Breathing is an important element of yoga and is an invisible extension of each pose. It is thought that the vital life force (or 'prana') enters the body with each breath. As with so much in Ayurveda, it also makes sense – if you hold your breath while exercising you are more likely to develop cramps. As a general rule try to enhale during movements that stretch the spine or open out the body. And inhale when you fold the body up, by bending or contracting your muscles. While you work, spread your fingers like the petals of a flower, and keep your movements as fluid as you can (this will become easier with time).

Yoga for Air types:

Your centre resides in your pelvis, so indulging in gentle stretching that stimulates the muscles of the pelvic area will soothe you.

The shoulder stand
The plough
The sun salutation (12 times slowly)

Yoga for Fire types:

The locust
The fish
The sun salutation (16 times moderately fast)

Yoga for Earth types:

As an Earth type, the centre of your energy resides in your chest. Therefore the following set of postures are particularly good for increasing circulation in your chest, and helping to prevent the onset of any Earth-type illnesses such as coughs and chest infections.

The tree
The plough
The sun salutation (12 times rapidly)

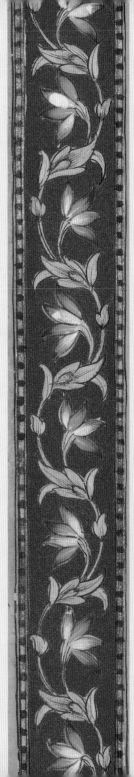

The Sun Salutation

This is a full body exercise that influences all the major joints and muscle groups and massages the internal organs. Aim to achieve each step as a fluid part of the whole without pauses between movements.

1. Stand tall, with your feet hip-width apart, and imagine an invisible string stretching upwards from your spine. Place your palms in a prayer position, resting lightly together in front of your chest with your elbows hanging by the side of your body. Close your eyes for a few moments while you become aware of yourself in the space and of your breathing and posture.

2. Take a deep breath as you stretch your arms out to your sides and whisk them outwards and upwards over your head. As you do this push your chest to the sky by bending the upper spine, but don't raise your shoulders or bend your waist.

3. Breathe out as you bend over, plunging your arms out to the sides and down to either side of your feet where your palms should rest parallel with your feet and flat to the floor. If you need to bend your knees to achieve this that is fine.

4. Breathe in as you push your right leg backwards and bend your left leg up under your chest, with your calf perpendicular to the floor, in a form of lunge where your face is tilted up to the sky. Concentrate on how long and straight your spine is. Try not to hunch your shoulders.

5. Breathe out as you push your left leg back behind you so both your feet are side by side, while you support yourself upon your hands. Push your bottom up to the sky making a shape like a pyramid. Relax your head and focus on the length of your neck.

6. Hold your breath as you lower your knees to the ground, but support yourself on your toes which should be curled under your feet to give

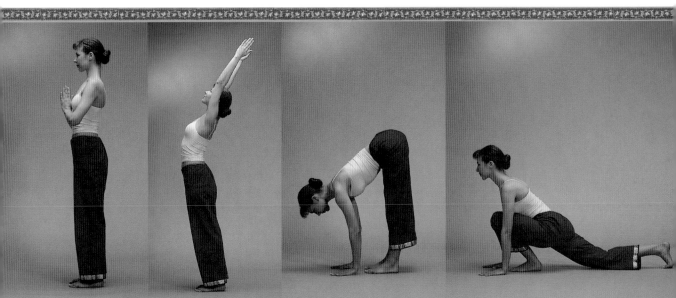

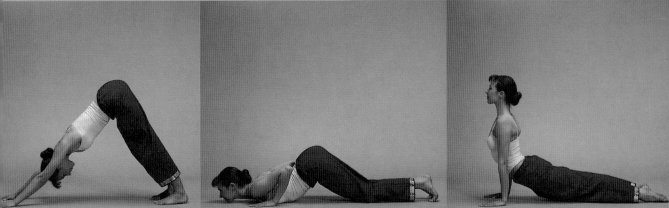

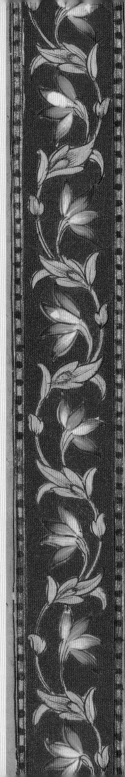

support. Then bend your arms as you gently lower your chest and chin to the floor, but keep your hips and bottom raised off the floor, so the only points of contact with the floor are your chin, chest, hands, knees and toes.

7. Breathe in as you push your upper body up like a cobra, supported on your hands, with your face and chest tilted upwards. Your hips are now dropped so your pelvis touches the floor. Ensure your shoulders are falling away from you, not held awkwardly.

8. Breathe out as you push yourself back into the pyramid position with both your feet side by side, your weight held on your hands, your head dropping down and your bottom pushed up to the sky.

9. Now lunge forward again, breathing in, and this time pushing your left leg forward with the calf perpendicular to the floor and your foot flat on the ground. Your right leg is bent at the knee, stretched out behind you and supported on its toes.

10. Breathe out as you step forward with your right leg, so you are standing on your feet, bent at the middle with your nose as near to your knees as possible and your palms flat on the ground either side of your feet. Bend your knees if you need to, don't strain your back.

11. Breathe in deeply as you stand up, pushing your arms up and out until your hands are above your head again. You can arch your upper spine backwards a little to enjoy this fully unfolded feeling and tilt your face and chest up towards the sky.

12. Breathe out as you gently bring your arms in a sweeping movement out from the sides of your body and into the prayer pose where your palms are lightly touching in front of your chest. Take a few deep breaths before repeating the cycle 11 times (don't worry, you can work up to this) alternating your starting leg each time. As you become familiar with the salutation pose it will flow into itself and you will begin to feel a buzz all over your body and suffused with the warm sensation of wellbeing.

The Postures (Asanas)

The locust

1. Lie on your tummy with your arms by your sides and your feet touching. Breathe in, and lift your right leg off the floor as high as it will go. Breathe out as you lower it to the floor.
2. Breathe in as you do the same with your left leg. Let yourself be led by your breathing and repeat this three times for each leg.
3. Now breathe in as you lift both legs off the floor a little way together and attempt to hold them there for a few seconds, before breathing out and bringing them back to the ground.

The shoulder stand

1. As you lie on your back, breathe out as you curl your knees towards you, and walk your hands up your back with your elbows taking the weight. Keep going until your torso is perpendicular to the floor, you are breathing out and your hands are holding onto the small of your back and your weight is supported on your shoulders. If you stretch your legs slightly over the top of your head and behind you, pointing your toes, you will be well balanced. Hold the movement for as long as possible, before beginning to breathe out as you gently uncurl your legs in a controlled way.

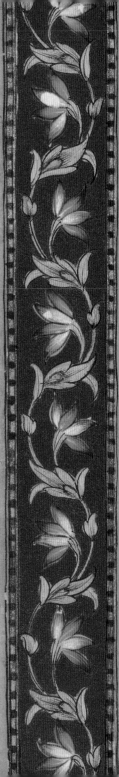

The plough

1. This is the same as the shoulder stand, but takes it one step further.
2. When you are in position with your toes pointing over your head, breathe in as you very slowly bring both legs over your head so your feet touch the floor behind you, breathing out as your toes touch down and curl to support the weight of your legs. You will be looking at your thighs as your hands drop away and your arms stretch out along the ground like two points of a star. Repeat three times, on the third repetition keep your toes against the floor as you take three deep breaths before unfurling.

The tree

1. Balance yourself by touching a table when performing this posture. Stand upright and breathe in while slowly bending your right knee until your heel is touching your left buttock.
2. Breathe out as you raise your arms in a straight line above your head and hold for as long as you can.
3. Then gently drop your right foot and arms and repeat on the other side. Do this three times for each side and you will begin to notice a marked improvement in the strength of your tummy muscles.

The fish

1. Lie on the floor with your arms by your sides and your legs straight in front of you. Breathe in as you arch your back so that the top of your head is in contact with the floor. Your back should lift off the floor so that the next point of support is your buttocks. Maintain the position while you breathe in and out deeply, before relaxing your spine and head back to the original supine position. Repeat three times.

Breathing Exercises

When you have finished your yoga practice you will probably be slightly out of breath. What better than to move into some meditative breathing exercises (known in traditional Ayurveda as 'pranayama'), both to refresh you and provide you with some concentrated focus for the day ahead. Ayurvedic breathing exercises improve creativity and help positive emotions to flow. As you breathe in during the exercise that I specify for each type, imagine that you are feeding your soul with the vital life force. Even if you do not believe this, such a positive visualization or affirmation has psychological benefits if you decide you want it to. You can use these techniques at any point during the day when you feel stressed out, tired, or in need of a moment to yourself. Traditionally these exercises are carried out while you are sitting cross-legged on the floor, but if you find this uncomfortable sit on a cushion, or even on a chair. You don't want any discomfort to detract from the benefits of focused breathing.

How to breathe

Unless we have exerted ourselves, we usually take only fairly shallow breaths that fill just the top part of the lungs. In fact, this isn't particularly good for us. When you take shallow breaths you stimulate nerves that are programmed to deal with a response to a stressful situation (when you are nervous you take very rapid shallow breaths as part of the fight or flight response) and this triggers the release of stress hormones, such as adrenaline, allowing us to quickly pump up our muscles if we are in danger so that we can escape.

Breathing basics:

Meditative breathing exercises known in traditional Ayurveda as 'pranayama' are refreshing and will help to provide you with some concentrated focus for the day ahead.

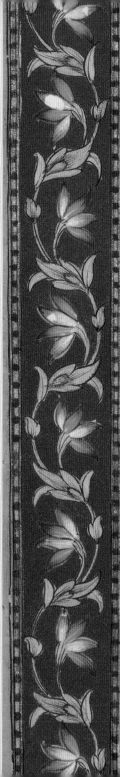

In contrast, the lower parts of the lungs contain nerves that soothe and calm us. This explains why our mothers instinctively suggest we 'take a deep breath' before a stressful activity. There are great benefits to be had from breathing deeply more of the time. By filling the whole lung with Air, you reduce anxiety, depression, nervousness, muscle tension and fatigue. Practising deep breathing also helps you get closer to an enviable place of mental clarity known as 'the alpha state'.

Sit or lie down in a comfortable position, with one hand resting lightly on your upper chest and the other on your abdomen. Breathe in and out slowly a few times and notice where the Air goes. Does your abdomen fill with Air first, or your chest? Does your chest or abdomen move alone?

Now breathe in slowly through your nose and direct your breath – you want to engorge your abdomen with Air first, by lowering your diaphragm. Imagine a balloon that you are filling with Air beneath the upper parts of your lungs.

Once your abdomen is swollen with Air, keep breathing in so that your chest also fills up and you feel it rise.

Breathe out, emptying your chest first, followed by your abdomen – breathing out shouldn't require any effort, just let it flow. Then repeat this deep breathing exercise, attempting to slow down your breathing so you create a rhythmic tide of Air entering and leaving your body.

Incorporate this new way of breathing into your daily lifestyle and you will feel much more refreshed and focused. And at the very least, do use it when you progress to the breathing exercises detailed below to gain maximum benefit.

Alternate nostril breaths – particularly suited to Air types. Repeat 12 times.

The left hemisphere of the brain is associated with male energy (it engages in logical thinking leading to scientific enquiry, judging, investigating, technology) and the right hemisphere with female energy (it uses lateral thinking to create intuitive thinking, compassion, art, poetry and love). We all have both elements in our brains, but some people have not learned how to access and use both sides equally.

The Ayurvedic Rishis discovered that our breathing patterns alter every hour or so. We breathe predominantly through one of our nostrils, before switching to the other. When we breathe through our right nostril we activate the left hemisphere of the brain (in the same manner that the right side of our body is governed by the left hemisphere) and vice versa.

The secret of this Ayurvedic breathing exercise is to harness and control the opposing male and female energies that flow through our nervous system. When yogis do alternate nostril breathing they believe that their male and female energies have become equally balanced (when in perfect balance they reach a form of enlightenment called '*brahman*', or pure awareness).

We can use alternate nostril breathing as a form of meditation and focus, giving clarity, focus and insight to our day.

Sit upright, either on a chair or in a cross-legged position on the floor. Your spine should be long and straight. Close your right nostril with the thumb on your right hand and breathe in deeply through your left nostril, taking care to fill the abdomen before the chest (see how to breathe, page 95). Hold your breath for a few moments, before using the ring and little finger of your right hand to close your left nostril so you breathe out through your right nostril. Then switch over using the thumb on your left hand to close your left nostril so that you breathe in deeply through your right nostril, before closing your right nostril with the ring and little fingers of your left hand. Repeat 12 times for each nostril.

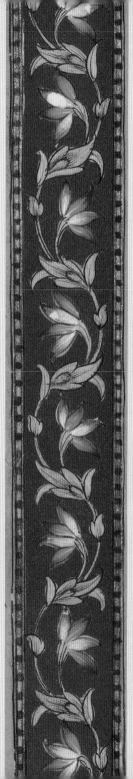

Fire breaths - particularly suited to Earth types - or for anyone who is feeling cold. Do one hundred of them.

Fire breathing helps to heat up the body, relieve asthma and increase the strength and capacity of the lungs. Sit upright and breathe in through your nose, keeping your mouth shut, and then exhale with some force. Begin to pick up inhalation and exhalation speed (you should sound a bit like a train picking up speed as it leaves a station). After you've done around thirty exhalations, take a minute's rest before continuing again.

Cooling breaths - particularly suited to Fire types - or for anyone who is feeling too hot. Do sixteen of them.

This is particularly helpful when you become over-heated. It helps to cool the entire body, relieves any burning in the eyes, throat or tongue, it also lowers the oral temperature, quenches thirst and is even believed to aid digestion. Simply curl your tongue into a tube and inhale slowly. This creates a sensation of cold. (If you can't curl your tongue, leave a tiny gap between your teeth, narrow your lips to a small hole and push your tongue against the back of your teeth before breathing in). Then swallow, and exhale normally through the nose, ensuring that the mouth stays shut. It's really surprisingly pleasant and effective.

Meditation basics:

Meditation is a way of bringing clarity and calm into your life.

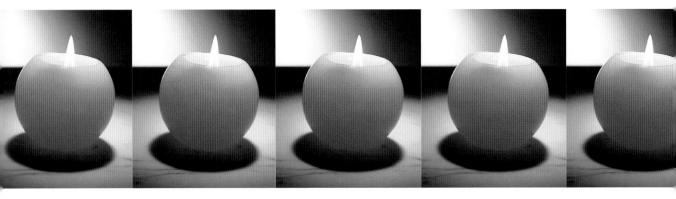

Meditation

We are always talking to ourselves. Not out loud, but in the cacophony of our minds. There is an ongoing dialogue which is usually so constant, persistent and insistent that we cease to notice it. It is like the background noise of a washing machine or busy road. It is only when the machine stops whirring or the cars go home at night that we notice the noise that was there before. But within our own minds we often do not have this opportunity to switch off the endless chattering. Thousands of years ago, the Ayurvedic teachers decreed that we are all 'the victims of memory'. How true this is. We exist against a backdrop of internalized fears, hopes, dreams, worries. And the truth is that we are controlled by these innermost perceptions. Should you take a risk or try something new? The answer you will choose tends to lie deep in your conditioning, your expectation, the inner voice that tells you whether or not you can achieve new goals. If you've had good experiences and have healthy self-esteem, your unspoken mind probably urges you on to happiness and future achievement, but perhaps makes it difficult to be satisfied with the reality of the moment. If you have failed in the past, been brought up with a lack of love or chosen friends who diminish your sense of self-worth, your internalized private voice probably limits you from going on to make the most of your potential. Either way it's time to find some space.

So, how to achieve this? Firstly, some misnomers. Meditation is not concentration, that takes effort and focus and it's tiring. Don't imagine that you have to say no to all thoughts, and banish all your mental activity. Meditation is a form of mental freedom. A way of finding yourself 'in the moment'. You do not deny what is going on around you – you hear, you smell, you think. But you do not linger. You do not judge, you do not process. You do not resist or invite. Gradually your mind becomes emptied of extraneous history. You notice not what your mind is telling you from experience, but only what is in the now.

Meditation basics:

Meditation is not concentration, that takes effort and focus and its tiring. It is a form of mental freedom.

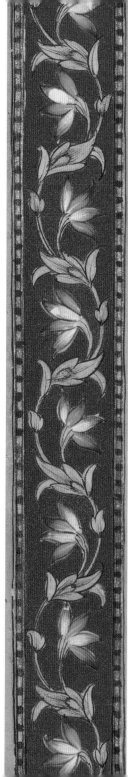

	Chakra	Effect
Air affirmation		
Yam	Heart	Increases love, compassion and stimulates the heart
Fire affirmation		
Ram	Solar Plexus	Increases digestive Fire, willpower and perception
Earth affirmation		
Vam	Lower abdomen	Reduces abdominal swelling due to water retention

Meditation is a way of learning to harness this intensely restorative awareness and being able to invest its clarity and calm into your life whenever you choose. This is not to say that you are so blissed out that you never get energized, passionate or suffused with action and creativity, but that you can do these things within a thoughtful and creative internal environment where there are no self-imposed limits, boundaries or self-limiting rules.

Mantra meditation encourages us to concentrate on one's personal affirmation or mantra, a simple but empowering phrase which is spoken aloud as a chant a number of times each day. This has the benefit of catching your attention on the sound, enabling your mind to 'transcend' the moment – for this reason it is sometimes called transcendental meditation (nothing to do with your teeth). Mantras are Sanskrit syllables, that were selected by the ancient Rishis after thousands of years of experimentation and practice, and they were chosen purely for the quality of the vibratory sound they create when uttered. The Bij mantras below do not actually have

Meditation helps to silence the mind.

any meaning, instead they are sounds that are believed to be particularly beneficial for the different types when they are in need of a lift.

How to use your mantra:

Close your eyes, sit comfortably and let your attention go to the appropriate chakra for your type. Repeat the mantra softly and at a relaxed pace, speaking aloud the mantra sound and letting it settle before speaking again. Focus on the quality of the sound and, each time you repeat it, let your voice become quieter and quieter until it is barely a whisper and finally just a thought. If you realize you are being distracted by external noise, or by your own thoughts, speak the mantra gently aloud again. Don't actively block out thoughts, that takes too much concentration, but just let them drift away. After five or six minutes (up to 15 if you prefer) keep your eyes closed and stay still for a couple of minutes. Imagine you are waking up from a deep sleep.

Empty bowl. This is an accessible and potentially powerful meditation – even when you are first practising it you will notice some benefit. Sit comfortably with your palms resting, loosely cupped and pointing upwards, on your knees. Open your mouth slightly and let your tongue rest on the roof of your mouth just behind your front teeth. Inhale and exhale normally, but let yourself become aware of the cool breath passing in through your nose and the warm breath passing back out again a few seconds later. For a few minutes imagine that you have shrunk into a tiny observer who is sitting inside your nostril, your hair ruffling in the warm and cool breezes that pass alternatively around you. Just let your lungs breathe naturally, don't force anything, just be very tiny and sit and feel the Air movements. Now follow your breath deeper. When you inhale follow the Air into the nose, to the back of the throat, past the trachea, into the top of the lungs, down through all the alveoli – the tiny pathways of the lungs that get smaller and smaller culminating in a series of

In Ayurveda silence is the birthplace of happiness.

cul de sacs down behind the belly button near the diaphragm when the lungs are full. When your breath reaches this final point you will sense a natural stop for a fraction of a second when you are neither breathing in or out (but don't exaggerate what happens naturally). Be aware of this stop and let yourself marvel at it. Then feel the exhalation begin and follow the breath back up in reverse until the Air passes back out from the nose and into the space in front of your face. Imagine it flowing out about nine inches in front of your eyes at the point when you feel a second natural stop, before the inhalation begins again. Keep your attention in that stop while it lasts.

These stops are the focus of the empty bowl meditation. Imagine that time stops in these two windows, and imagine that when time stops mind stops and you are free from everything – competitiveness, jealousy, worry, fear, concern and stress. View the stop as a doorway to pure consciousness and positive emotion. If you are full of negative thinking there is no room for peace, but these small doorways are places of great tranquillity.

If you practise this meditation for 10 to 15 minutes in the morning and evening you will gradually find your awareness of the time in the stops increases and, as the name suggests, you – the empty bowl – can be filled with positivity and calm.

So-hum. This is very similar to the Empty Bowl Meditation as we sit and become aware of our breath. But in this case imagine the word *So* as you breathe in, and the word *Hum* as you speak out. Don't speak them aloud however. The Rishis believed that inhaling symbolizes living, while exhaling symbolizes dying. A baby breathes in at birth, when someone dies she or he literally 'expires' as the final breath passes out. As you say So (which means 'the divine') you are breathing in life, and, as you follow it with Hum (which means 'ego') you are exhaling ego and limitation. At its most extreme this meditation is said to lead you to union with the cosmic consciousness as your mind empties itself entirely. Even if you do not experience such a profound effect, the So-hum meditation should certainly lower your heart rate and help re-energize you.

Mindfulness

Why not try this form of 'wakeful' meditation which you can do any time, any place. Watching your thinking in the simple ways described below gives you a new perspective and invigorates your inner life.

Air types are often inspired thinkers with rapid, fertile minds, but when under stress or out of balance those thoughts can accelerate, becoming chaotic and unconstructive. If you are under slightly more stress than usual, you can benefit enormously from taking a mental step backwards and listening, almost as an outsider, to the melee of different thoughts that go by.

Fire types have discerning personalities, but can become overtly judgmental. Whenever you notice you are thinking overly discriminating thoughts meditate on the thoughts and become 'mindful' of the pattern of your less positive mindset. Concentrate on thinking the opposite of your judgements even if you disagree with them, just to remind yourself there is always another perspective.

Earth types have a more placid outlook and are steady, reliable thinkers. This can be a gift in times of turmoil, but can lapse into adapting less to new circumstance than is beneficial, or obsessing about the same thought endlessly. If you sense you are creeping into this pattern become mindful of what you are doing, this in itself will stimulate fresh ideas and kick-start your thinking into a fresh direction.

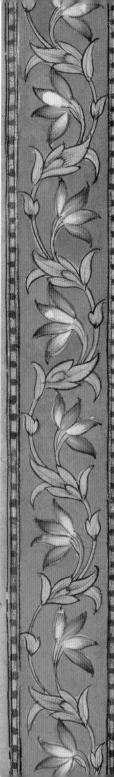

Body purification

Opposites are said to attract. In fact, countless relationship studies undermine this maxim. However, when it comes to our relationship with our own body the mantra does have authority. Keeping our bodies in balance can be a tricky process and you will need to indulge in some lifestyle and diet tweaking. Here, the Ayurvedic rule of thumb is to apply the opposite type or quality to fine-tune your system: If you are agitated or distressed, then sit down quietly and meditate for a while; if you are feeling chilly, sip some warming soup or make a cup of tea; and if you are feeling tense and hot, the best way to care for yourself is to have a cool bath, eat some fruit fresh from the fridge or treat yourself to some ice-cream. This makes so much sense that it's amazing we don't automatically think of this 'yin/yang' style solution to life's smaller ills as the right panacea always.

The truth is that we often don't have the time and, unfortunately, toxins and imbalances can then build up to levels that require a more intense approach. Fortunately, Ayurveda is big on purification. There are many good practitioners who can help take the matter out of your hands, and a visit to a clinic or spa embracing Ayurvedic practices can also be a wonderful treat. But the good news is that it is also possible to turn your own home into an Ayurvedic sanctuary, where your bathroom is re-cast as a temple to the senses and your bedroom as a restorative cocoon. Follow the advice below for the theory, and kitchen-cupboard solutions for effective external and internal detoxification programme I endorse.

Purification helps to eliminate toxins and

External Detoxification
Massage With Oils (*Purvakarma*)

The starting point for the wonderful range of Ayurvedic physical therapy is a detoxifying massage. A unique combination of oils and herbs are carefully selected and blended to either stimulate and energize or soothe the body, while encouraging toxins to rise to the surface. This is a great place to start your Ayurvedic detoxification ritual. Massage is wonderful, to receive and to give. It relaxes you while imparting your skin with beneficial oils. Ayurveda views the skin like a second mouth and what better to charm its palate with than the benefits of the ultimate exercise in tactility. Ayurvedic purists would probably overlook these sensory benefits; massage is a serious business, but it's also completely delicious.

Dosha Balancing Kit

Ayurvedic massage is particularly effective because, rather than using a generic oil for everyone, there are massage oils geared to perfection for each type which have been formulated and handed down over the millennia. The right massage oil for your type will nourish your skin, reduce fatigue and stress, improve metabolism, slow the effects of ageing, while adding lustre to the skin and hair. It also helps to rejuvenate the body by detoxification and promotes a sense of tranquillity and wellbeing.

Air (vata) types should use calming oils: sesame, olive, almond, wheat germ and castor oils.

Fire (pitta) types should use cooling oils: sunflower, almond, coconut and sandalwood oils.

Earth (kapha) types should use invigorating oils: mustard, corn oil or canola oil.

Purification basics:

Massage is a wonderful way to begin any Ayurvedic detoxification process.

imbalances within the body which may build up over time.

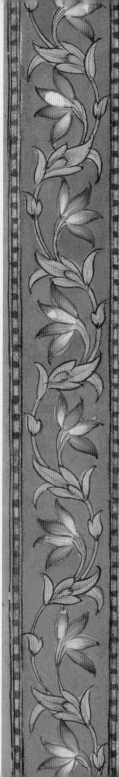

How to Use Your Custom Oil

Choose a five day period – perhaps when you are on holiday or have a week fairly free at home. Warm half a cup (take care it is not too hot) of your favoured oil – NB never boil the oil as this changes its properties, either heat in a microwave or indirectly and, while standing in the bath, massage it all over your body. Let the embalming softness soothe you as you rub it in well from head to toe. Spend a minimum of fifteen minutes anointing yourself with the warm unguent in this way. When the oil is thoroughly absorbed, turn on the shower and blast your skin with hot water. You can wash with Ayurvedic neem soap – but don't remove all the oil from your skin. Instead try this ancient Ayurvedic technique known as an *Ubvartan Scrub*.

Ubvartan Scrub

Take a handful of chickpea flour (or porridge oats if you don't have it to hand) and make looping massaging motions over your skin to slough off any dead cells and absorb the oil. Beware your plumbing: You'll need to flush the drains with plenty of hot water to prevent spontaneous chappatis! This process is also wonderful after sweat treatments.

Aromatherapy

What bliss! Those fabulous essential oils were discovered by Ayurvedic doctors to pacify aggravated patients. Essential oils are highly volatile aromatic oils produced by plants in order to attract insects and fight off disease. When our brain detects molecules of these oils we experience a powerful response that subconsciously influences our memory, emotions and libido.

Using aromatherapy oils in Ayurvedic massage follows the opposites attract theory. You calm an inflamed Fire type with cooling oils; you reinvigorate a sluggish Earth type with a stimulating oil; you soothe stress for Air types with a calming balm.

Air types: Use ylang-ylang, patchouli, geranium, lavender, cedar wood and myrrh.

Earth types: Use frankincense, sage, rosemary, camphor, basil and eucalyptus.

Fire types: Use saffron, jasmine, rose, sandalwood, gardenia and lotus.

Massage techniques

Friction Massage

Earth types: This is particularly good for you as you are prone to suffer cold extremeties. However, use in the morning only to energize yourself and do not exceed using this technique twice a week to avoid over oiling the skin.

Air types: Use the same technique with a lighter touch but massage more frequently to help ground yourself in physical sensation.

Fire types: Heat the oil to a lower temperature to avoid aggravating the skin. Sensitive skin types also generally require less frequent massage and will benefit from massage in the afternoon when Fire can be running high.

This is a wonderful stimulating massage using a simple friction technique which will really set those nerve endings zinging. As all your nerves ultimately end within your brain this is a massage to enervate and energize. Ayurvedic massage does not tend to involve deep muscle massage, instead it aims to stimulate subtler energies. The touch should be light but firm, but how much pressure depends on your type:

Dry skin (Air) types: Use a 'Sattvic' touch, that is light, calm and slow. Too much pressure aggravates Air types and will lead to feelings of unsettled agitation.

Sensitive skin (Fire) types: Use a 'Rajasic' touch, moderate pressure and speed but not too much so firey types are not aggravated.

Oily skin (Earth) types: Use a 'Tamasic' touch, this is deep and vigorous and ensures stimulation for the slower Earth natures.

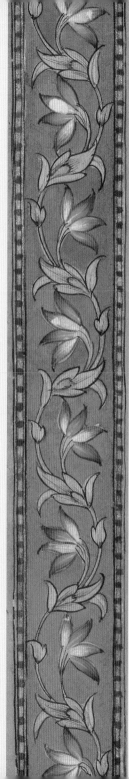

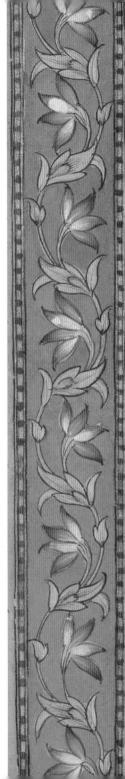

The friction technique produces heat which awakens the skin and warms the oil, allowing it to disperse all over the body so it is absorbed more quickly.

1. Warm the appropriate oil for your type (if you do not have it to hand any type can use almond oil as this is quite neutral and will not imbalance or otherwise affect your doshic type). Heat up at least half a cup in a microwave or in a waterbath, but you can use more. The more oil you use the greater the benefit.

2. Choose which area of your body, or your partner's body, you wish to treat. This technique is particularly helpful to warm cold extremities – such as legs, face, hands or feet. Earth types are particularly prone to feeling cold in these areas, but the massage has benefits for everyone. Pour a generous amount of warmed oil over the area to be treated.

3. Use both your hands on their side, rolling them around in a circular motion towards you like a bicycle wheel turning. This should be as rapid as possible to achieve the full benefits. The strokes should be swift and firm, but not hard. Only the side of your little fingers and the side of your palm should come into contact with the skin being treated.

4. Gradually move the bicycle wheel around the area being treated. The best benefits are achieved after five minutes.

5. After the treatment the area massaged will still be very oily. Wrap the area in a towel and sit back while the nourishing oil is absorbed into your skin. This takes a minimum of half an hour.

If you have friction massage as a full body treatment in my clinic you will benefit from two therapists working on you simultaneously. During a normal massage only one therapist works on the body which tends to activate the opposite side of your brain. The benefit of two masseurs – as well as being a hedonistic indulgent – is so that both sides of the brain are stimulated equally at the same time.

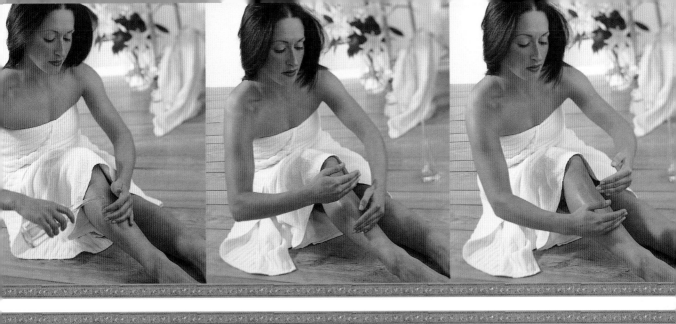
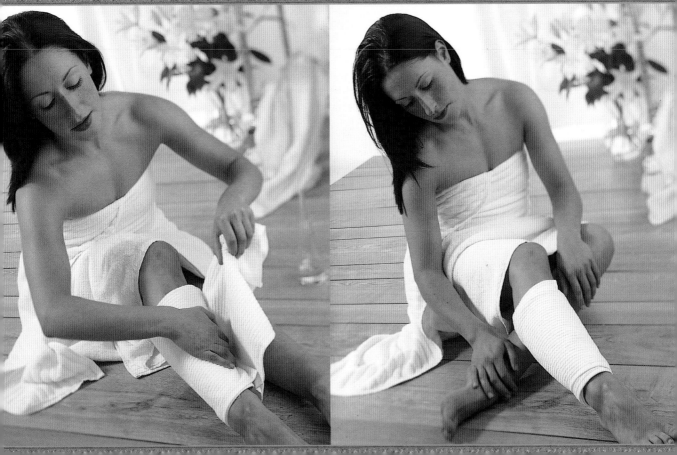

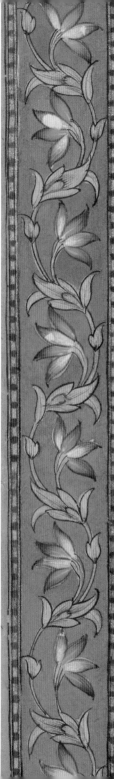

Scalp Massage

This is a very relaxing massage – particularly good if you should choose to give it to a partner. It is nourishing for scalp and hair, encouraging new growth and stimulating your brain.

1. Locate your '*Brahma Randhra*' – the middle of the scalp about ten finger widths above the eyebrows. This was the part of the skull that did not form fully until after infancy. Ayurveda believes this is the seat of bliss where the lifeforce '*prana*' enters the body. Massaging this point is a good way to relieve tension headaches.

2. Press your fingers firmly into the visual centre at the nape of the neck 'the *Manya Mula*'. Pat the point, applying light pressure. Massage it clockwise using your middle finger. Then wind a section of hair growing from this point around your finger and pull firmly to stimulate the scalp. Good for relieving tension headaches.

3. Press your fingers onto the crown or '*Adhipati*' chakra at the back of the top of the head between the ears. Pat the point, then massage clockwise before winding a section of hair and pulling. Good for relieving hypertension.

4. Comb your hair and make furrowed partings into which you pour quite generous amounts of the heated oil appropriate for your type. Massage the oil firmly and slowly into your skin as if washing deeply with shampoo in low motion.

5. Part a new area of the head and repeat until the entire scalp has been treated.

6. If you are preparing to sleep or suffering from insomnia spend some time massaging both temples with a fairly firm pressure.

7. Let the oil nourish your hair for a minimum of one hour. Then wash in the normal way.

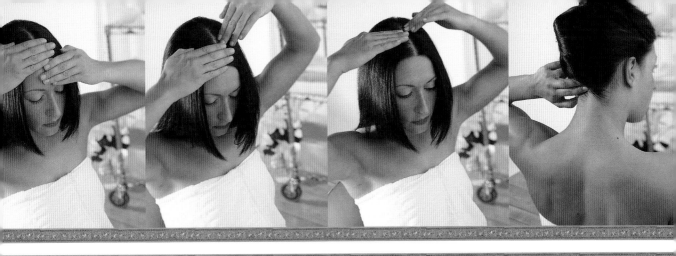

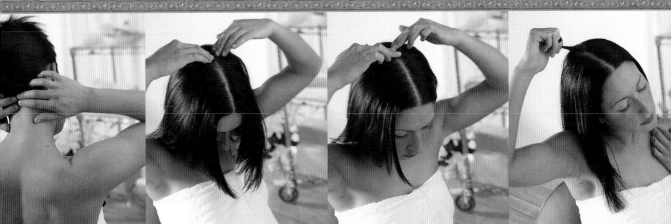

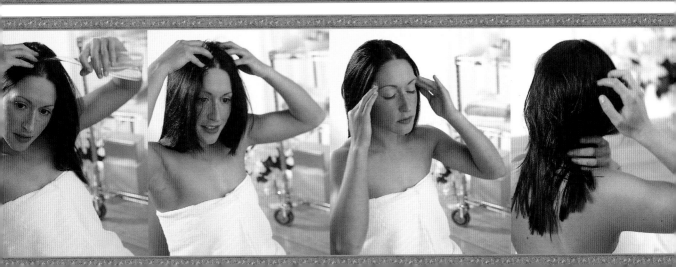

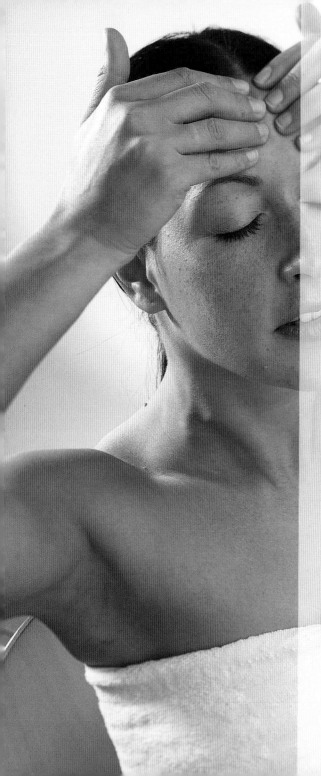

Face Massage

Use the appropriate face oil for your type. This is a great massage at any time of the day.

1. Using both palms gently massage your neck upwards from bottom to top.
2. Place your index finger in the space between chin and lower lip. Place your middle finger under your chin. Using a firm pressure on the jawbone massage all the way from chin to jawline near the ear. This stimulates the marma point known as 'Hanu'.
3. Laugh lines and cheeks. Massage your laugh lines firmly in an upwards direction with your index fingers. Be firm and precise, be aware of the underlying muscles of the face that you are stimulating. When you reach the nose continue out across the apple shaped area of the cheeks.
4. Point the ring fingers of both hands at the point just under your eyebrows and push firmly, inching your way along the brow bone and then around your eye as is drawing a circle. This is surprisingly enervating.
5. The sixth chakra, known as 'the third eye', is located in the centre of the forehead between and above the eyes. Place your index finger upon it and massage repeatedly.
6. Place all eight fingers upon your forehead and massage to help decrease wrinkles.

Following a massage, always allow yourself time to rest and recuperate for a while to enjoy the full benefit of this refreshing therapy.

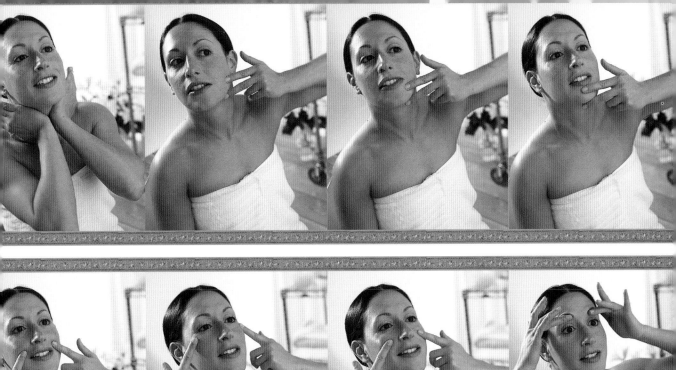

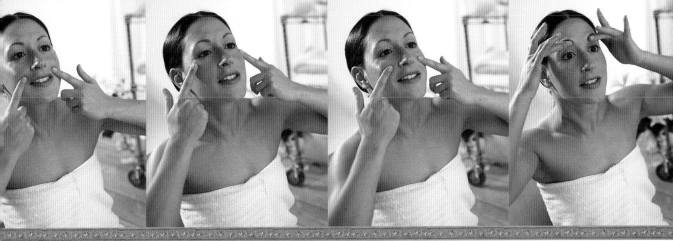

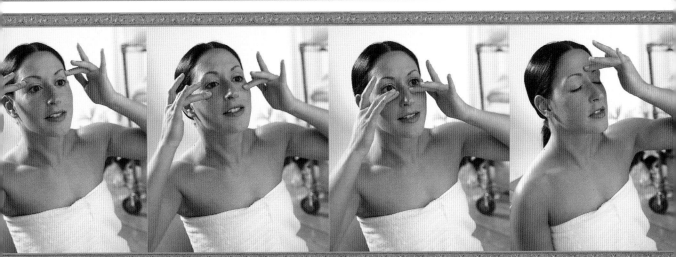

Emergency Weekend Kit

Make one weekend a month a mini Ayurvedic cleansing celebration. Embrace the guidelines below and return to work on Monday a calmer, refreshed, more uplifted soul:

- Drink boiled water with herbs infused in it instead of stimulants such as tea and coffee. Add peppermint or coriander, or at the very least use shop-bought tisanes.
- Avoid alcohol, cigarettes and processed food.
- Wear loose, comfortable light clothes.
- Think invigorating walks rather than extreme exercise.
- Splash out on organic vegetables and fruit; eat simply but well.
- Turn off the television, and seek your stimulation from reading, conversation, painting or quiet contemplation.
- Make sure you sleep for at least nine hours.
- Have frequent warm baths.
- Pamper yourself with candles, aromatherapy oils, incense and soothing music.
- Treat yourself to a divine bath of the five nectars. A bath is a rejuvenating exercise for mind as well as body and in the Vedic tradition the ultimate bath soak consists of the five nectars. These foods – milk, honey, yoghurt, ghee and banana – are considered by Ayurveda to be the five perfect foods. It's so simple to worship the temple of your body in this way, as the Rishis used to worship the temple statues. All you need to do is combine the mashed pulp of a banana with two tablespoons of milk, one teaspoonful of honey, one teaspoon of yoghurt, and one of ghee. Massage the sweet-scented mix onto your skin and plunge into a warm bath to nourish, soften, smooth and re-energize your skin. Could anything be more perfect?

Sweat Therapy (*Swedana Karma*)

After an effective massage the surface of your skin will be swimming in expelled toxins and you need to sweat them out. In Western culture, sweating is rather frowned upon. I remember hearing an English phrase that perfectly summed this up: 'Only horses sweat – men perspire and women merely glow.' That may have been how Victorian gentlemen preferred to view the world, but fortunately things have changed. The steam bath is a now a common fixture of the gym but Ayurveda with its earthy, sensual worship of the body's natural function takes this a step further. Swedana, or sweating, is the second part of the two-step preparation for Panchakarma.

Sweating helps you to detoxify by promoting the elimination of waste by stimulating the sweat glands. It also warms up the muscles, helps relieve heaviness due to bloating, encourages the elimination of disease and improves the lustre and condition of your skin – notice how soft and fresh your face looks after a sauna. In strict Ayurveda, the practitioner may apply heated gauze, towels and bandages to the patient's body. Warm pastes may be used in order to baste pain and swelling (much like seaweed wraps and treatments in the West). Rice, sand, salt and mixed herbs are sometimes heated, pushed into gauze bags and used to encourage sweating by application to specific areas. Sometimes medicinal leaves are infused with hot water and added to sugar to create a sweaty sweet bath.

Similar effects can be achieved with any sweating method; physical exertion, body wraps, dry heat sweating (sauna) or wet heat sweating (steam room). If you don't feel like going for a jog and don't have access to a gym, create your own home spa using herbalized steam to stimulate the elimination of toxins through the skin.

Home Steam Bath

Fill the bath with hot water and add a few drops of the herb that suits your skin type before closing the shower curtains to encase the steam. Add cold

Massage basics:

After a massage always allow yourself time to rest and recuperate and to enjoy the full benefit of this therapy.

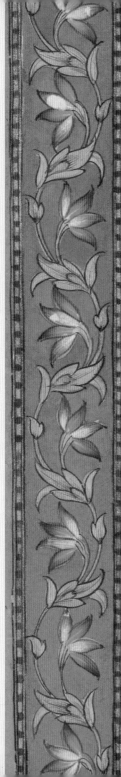

water to your preference and soak for five to 10 minutes in the vapours until your body and face begin to sweat. Then rinse.

Oily (Earth) skin: Sage or rosemary.

Dry (Air) skin: Bala or dashamala.

Sensitive (Fire) skin: Camomile or comfrey.

Bed Simmering

After your steam bath, or in place of it if you prefer, try a dry heat approach. Heat several soft towels in a linen cupboard or over a heated towel rail. Wrap yourself up in them and plunge into bed beneath a thick duvet or several blankets for the ultimate cook-in-towelling experience. Give yourself 10 minutes to sweat warmly and copiously, then whip off the towels and push them into the washer as you dash under a nice cooling shower. Then you can treat yourself to a nice re-balancing and exfoliating Ubvartan scrub (see page 106).

Internal Detoxification - *Panchakarma*

You owe it to yourself to reward yourself with a life in balance. What better way to achieve this than with a blissful session of Panchakarma – the indulgent central tenet of the Ayurvedan philosophy that traditionally follows on from the external preparation above. This is the process of internal purification, the ultimate system of 'inner cleansing' which gives you the power, knowledge and right to treat your body – that hardworking, slavish, often exhausted vehicle – as a temple. You can go overboard here. Take a trip to an Indian supermarket, or specialist Ayurvedic centre, and have a razzle. Invest in some of the herbs and preparations I am discussing, buy some pretty glass jars with cork lids to store them, and set aside a shelf in your bathroom – this will become your easy access Ayurveda rejuvenative and restorative zone.

Traditionally, Panchakarma (which means literally 'five actions') is a vigorous multi-step process of internal detoxification. Although the more extreme forms of the treatment are only available under the guidance of a practitioner in a clinic, some of the steps also have home versions which I present below.

The value of Panchakarma is the way it helps to dislodge and flush toxins from our bodies using the organs of elimination that the body uses naturally. Ayurveda is deliciously earthy. You are actively encouraged to express wind, belch, analyze your eliminations, and generally enjoy the natural functions of your body. You may not want to do all this under the watchful eye of an Ayurvedic clinician, but you can do what you like in the privacy of your own home. And there is good reason for encouraging these natural processes of elimination. Most diseases travel with us for some time, developing slowly like a snowball rolling across a lawn — we gradually accumulate throughout our lives the triggers for the major diseases of the Western world; arthritis, osteo-porosis, diabetes, cancer and heart disease. Helping flush away the toxins that lead to these disorders can help avoid their onset.

Seasonal changes exert challenges upon our constitutions and this is why Panchakarma is best performed with each change of season. Ideally, the Ayurvedic clinics suggest you spend nine or 10 days re-adjusting to each sea-sonal variation. Therefore the best time to create your own Panchakarma spa is for a minimum of two or three days at the beginning of spring, summer, and winter (autumn is not recognized as a true season in Ayurvedic terms, but that's not to stop you enjoying Panchakarma as summer merges into autumn). Even if you do not attend to your Ayurvedic ritual at any other time, why not use this great excuse to treat yourself to at least three pampering weekends each year? And why spend money and time when, with the knowledge you will learn below, you will be able to create your own Ayurvedic sanctuary behind familiar doors — it's even more fun with a friend.

Why is Internal Cleansing so Beneficial?

When you over stress your body's internal systems with an unhealthy diet, neg-ative feelings, late nights, overwork, and excess stimulants, Ayurvedic teaching suggests that the body's biological Fire ('*agni*') becomes weakened. Food begins

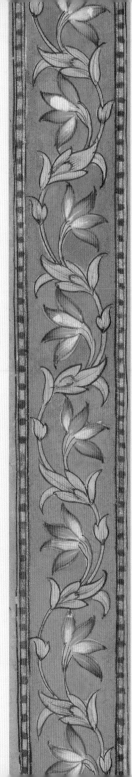

to be poorly digested and the un-absorbed food particles clump together to form a sticky unhealthy toxicity (known as 'ama'). Gradually, this filters into the intestines and meanders through the blood vessels infusing the tissue and muscle mass with toxic lethargy. When ama lodges there over time, the body is forced to fight through this barrier of sludge to function normally, and disease is more likely to begin its early stages of incubation. Traditional Ayurveda understands disease as 'a crisis of ama' in which the body is struggling to eliminate the accumulation of all that toxicity. In more familiar Western terms, you can envisage ama as the feeling of lethargy and heaviness you feel when you have been working too hard, eating too many heavy processed meals, not getting enough fresh Air and generally not respecting your system. Your breath might become rather pungent, your head muddled and aching, your back may be stiff, you may have constipation and excess gas along with a bad taste in the mouth. If you've got a thick coating on the tongue, you've got excess ama and you need to work fast to help eliminate the disease-forming toxins.

The Importance of Water

No mention of holistic methods for flushing out diseases would be complete without mention of water. We have evolved around this life-giving fluid and drinking six to eight glasses of tap water a day is really the best way of ensuring that your digestive flow keeps moving and your body is purified internally as well as externally. If you drink water you allow your body to work with substances that are at lower concentration, giving plenty of liquidic legroom for everything to function as it should. The remarkable thing is just how well our bodies function superficially despite being dehydrated, but you owe it to yourself to give your overworked organs as much respite as you can by guzzling as much water as you can manage. If you need to make it a little more palatable, twist a slice of lemon or lime into a jug of water and store it in the fridge before decanting into ice-filled glasses. Lecture over!

Only trained clinicians can offer the complete re-balancing system of

Purification basics:

Drinking six to eight glasses of water daily is the best way to ensure your digestive flow keeps moving and your body is purified internally as well as externally.

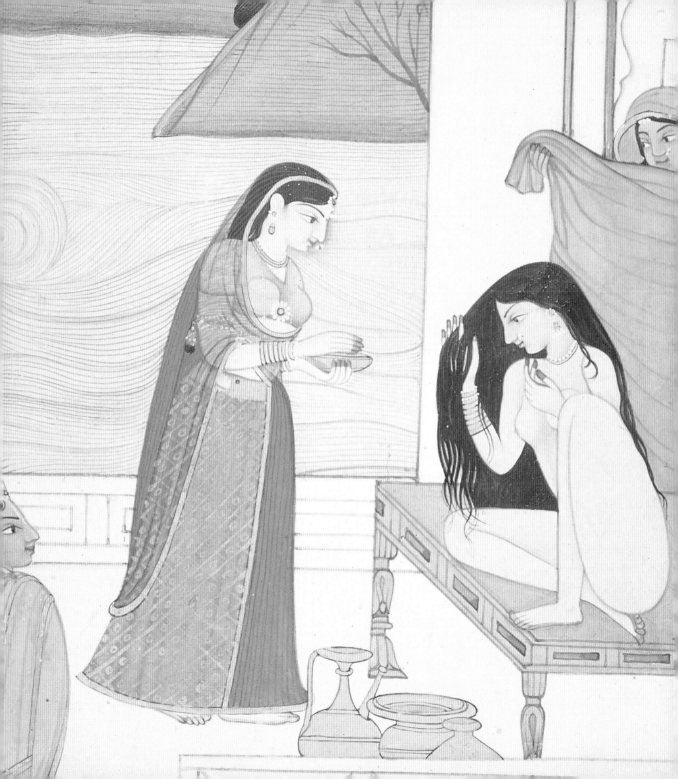

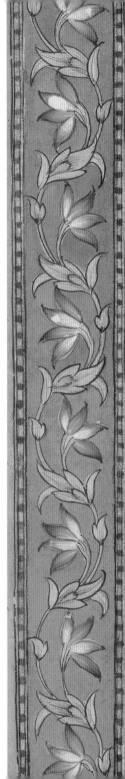

Panchakarma. However, elements of this restorative therapy can be completed usefully at home. There are five steps, four of which can be used in a modified form at home – although you might view them as a bit extreme for anything other than the experience of the experience. In that case, stick to the massages.

A. Gentle Purging (*Virchana*)

During your Ayurvedic treatment period drink half a teaspoon of triphala steeped in half a cup of boiling water. This herb is a safe, mild but effective laxative which will encourage any clogging in your digestive tract to be flushed through. Eliminating toxins in this way is a process that I encourage, but don't worry if it's not for you. Just try to increase your intake of water so that the concentrations of toxins are weakened and flushed out in your urine instead.

B. Internal Balancing

If you are feeling daring, you might like to experiment with an Ayurvedic medicated enema ('*basti*') after you have bathed. If this doesn't appeal to you, that's fine but if you follow these instructions you can try this interesting therapy in the comfort of your home. There are claims that this is a particularly effective treatment for Air related disorders including fever and hyperacidity, but you should avoid basti if you are pregnant, or are suffering the symptoms of diarrhoea, indigestion, breathlessness, any rectal disorders, or haemorrhoids.

Wait at least three hours after eating and make a nest of towels on the downstairs bathroom floor (it helps to be near the kitchen so you can heat your ingredients without travelling miles). You will need to buy an enema bag or syringe from a chemist and read the instructions. Warm quarter of a cup of sesame oil and introduce it internally, holding on to it for about 10 minutes, but keep it inside while you introduce the next stage. This oil enema is also wonderful for your skin; the colon is an important part of the absorption process for the nutrients in our food and the oil from an enema is absorbed effortlessly into the system, lubricating the skin from the inside out.

Earlier, you will have prepared two tablespoons of dashamoola in a pint of water to make a rich looking tea. When it has cooled down, strain it and introduce it internally. Hold on to the liquid for as long as you feel comfortable, about 25 minutes is good – and don't worry if it disappears! If you are dehydrated, as we frequently are in the West, you may absorb most of the herbal tea. This is absolutely normal and perfectly safe.

When you have held onto the liquid for as long as suggested, or until you feel ready to end the session, sit upon the loo and let the enema fluids and any material leave your system.

C. Nasal Scenting

Stand by for a rather extraordinary fact and bear it in mind next time you wander through that city street: Allergists believe we inhale two and half tablespoons of solid particles each day – more in cities. These include pollen, car exhaust and fumes. We have good filtration processes thanks to the tiny hairs that line the inside of our noses and which continually comb the Air we breathe, much like a whale draining the sea for plankton. But our sinuses and the delicate tissues responsible for processing our sense of smell continue to be bombarded.

To give them some loving care you can't beat this quick fix tip known in Ayurveda as 'Nasya': Use an eyedropper or the tip of your little finger to introduce two drops of sesame oil into your nose. Lightly massage the inside of your nostril before throwing your head back and inhaling sharply three or four times so that the oil is carried high into your nasal passages.

D. The Heavenly Compress (Shirodhara)

Imagine basking on a treatment bed. The lights are low, the music inducing a state of soporific calm. Your hands and feet are warm, and you are swaddled in towels. Upon your forehead the most delectable magic-carpet ride is occurring minute after minute as you drift and dream, beguiled by the

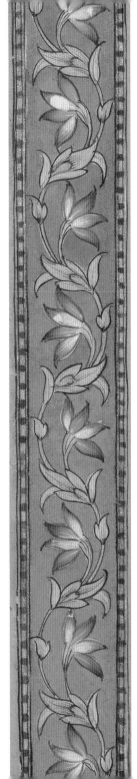

soothing warm sensations running through your hair line. A steady stream of medicated oil is pouring in a needle-thin trickle upon the middle of your forehead. The oil runs over your temples, down through your hair and out into a special drainage hole under your head. This is massage of the third eye – known in Ayurveda as shirodhara. As you lay there, you won't want to be troubled with the details, only with the restorative sensations, but this is one of the most powerful Ayurvedic treatments – designed to relieve mental tensions and induce a heavenly state of mind – and well worth a try. I'm waiting for it to catch on at the country's leading health farms where Indian head massage is already popular.

Great stuff ... but not very practical for your home spa. However, you can benefit from a smaller-scale massage of the third eye (the 'chakra' or energy centre that is located in the middle of your forehead) by using a heavenly compress. It should follow a self-massage and steam bath after which your mind and body will be more receptive. All you need to do is soak a cloth in the oil that is appropriate to your type, place it on your third eye and lie back with eyes closed for ten minutes. The effect can be enhanced by burning incense and playing music. Oh yes, and do switch off the chattering mind!

Air types: use warm sesame oil.

Fire types: use equal parts of cool milk and coconut oil and perhaps a few drops of rose water.

Earth types: warm sesame oil and ginger tea in equal proportions.

The Fifth Element

The final component of the traditional Ayurvedic cleansing treatment is known as 'emetic vomiting'. The Rishis believed that drinking noxious tasting concoctions with plenty of water to stimulate the vomiting response could be beneficial. While it might be useful if you have swallowed something bad or poisonous, it is considered in our culture to be inadvisable with its overtones of bulimia and therefore I do not recommend it.

Extra Panchakarma Cleansing Options

In addition to the primary therapies, Panchakarma includes other inner cleansing treatments which can be used according to an individual's needs to achieve body purification:

Oleation

We massage our skin, the second mouth, with oils. Likewise, an internal massage can help to flush out toxins. All you need to do is melt two dessert spoonfuls of ghee and swallow them each morning for three days. (To make ghee: simmer butter for 15 minutes until the whitish curds that form at the bottom of the pan begin to turn a golden colour as the water boils off from the butter. Then simply drain off the liquid ghee above and leave to cool in a tub).

NB: Do not drink ghee if you have high cholesterol levels – your doctor can advise. If you have high levels substitute flaxseed oil for ghee as it will do the trick while helping to reduce cholesterol levels.

Air types: add a pinch of rock salt

Earth types: add a tiny pinch of ginger and one of black pepper

Fire types: benefit from ghee with nothing added.

Ayurvedic Tonics

You can give your cells a special treat by fuelling them with an Ayurvedic rejuvenative depending on your type:

Air types: mix a teaspoon of ashwagandha in a cup of hot milk each morning and evening.

Fire types: mix a teaspoon of shatavari in a cup of warm milk each morning and evening.

Earth types: mix a teaspoon of punarnava in a cup of warm water each morning and evening.

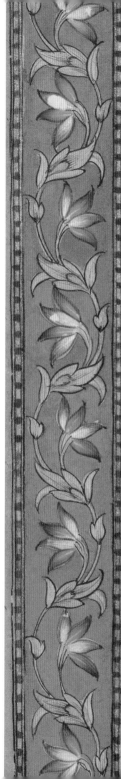

Sexuality

Imagine a Vedic sage and you probably imagine a wizened hermit living a celibate life on a hilltop contemplating his navel, eschewing women and seeking enlightenment. You certainly do not envisage a loving married man with a wife and a brood of children. Yet the philosophers who devised Ayurveda often married and had families. Ayurveda believes that the expression of our sexual desires is a wonderful part of life and is a vital natural element of enhancing spirituality when practised with a partner whom we love. Enjoying sex for pleasure within a marriage has been promoted in Vedic texts since the Kama Sutra.

Good sex is considered by Ayurveda to improve the bond between husband and wife, and indeed this element of your life has the potential to create enormous pleasure, encourage stress release, and offer satisfaction using the wonderful tools of both your bodies and your minds. This is because sexual energy (or what is known in Ayurveda as 'prana') is our life essence. To suppress it – and equally to overuse it – damages our ability to experience the best that life has to offer. If you suppress or cut off your sexuality, you are literally cutting off the life force. Taken to its extreme, Ayurveda suggests that complete abstinence can be a way of negatively cutting yourself off from life. Sex is a natural function of the body and Ayurveda stresses that it is necessary for complete holistic health. What's more, it is a great form of exercise, and it also relieves stress and tension.

Ayurveda believes that the expression of

Ayurveda makes some particularly interesting suggestions about the role of this potentially tremendous creative force in our lives. Initially, it suggests that our type influences the frequency of sexual activity we should be indulging in. Strict Ayurveda suggests that although an Earth type can make love two or three times a week because they have a strong constitution, the more fragile Air types should abstain other than once or twice a month. Fire types are said to be able to thrive on making love once every two weeks. These recommendations, although perhaps appropriate for some people, are generally insufficient for the sexual appetites we are encouraged to enjoy in the West, and take little account of different types who are happily married to each other. The point here is not to slavishly follow this advice, or change your own relationship in any way if you are both happy with it, but to understand what lies behind these suggestions.

In much of the Indian sub-continent and especially within Ayurvedic teaching, there is a belief that making love too frequently reduces your vital energy – or 'oja'. You experience this as a couple when you nestle against one another and fall off to sleep after you have made love. There is a biological reason for this – the sperm is more likely to find the egg if the woman stays lying down, and she is more likely to stay lying down if her partner is too – but additionally, Ayurvedic teaching suggests that this reduction in energy, if practised too frequently, leaves us fundamentally weakened and more vulnerable to picking up stray bugs. The point is, if you are going to have a more active relationship than suggested by the Vedic texts, my advice is to take a few simple, commonsense steps to ensure that you are not being depleted in this way.

Because of the delicious sleepy state created by love-making, Ayurvedic teaching suggests that the ideal time to make love is between 10 and 11pm. Although a man's sex drive is at its peak in the morning, it

Bedroom basics:

Sex is a natural function of the body and Ayurveda stresses that it is necessary for complete holistic health. What's more, it is a great form of exercise, and it also relieves stress and tension.

our sexual desires is a wonderful and vital part of life.

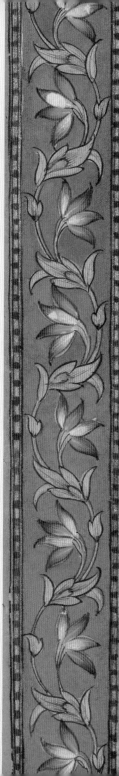

is better to use this vitality to face the challenges of the day ahead. If you do make love in the morning, try and leave time to offer each other a quick restorative massage to encourage your energy to wake up again. Some Ayurvedic sages recommend drinking delicious tasting almond milk to invigorate yourself in the morning if you have just made love (before going to bed the night before soak 10 raw almonds in water, peel off the skins and blend them in the morning along with a pinch of nutmeg, saffron and ginger, then add a cup of warm milk).

Creating a sexual life that satisfies both partners is also often misunderstood in the West. The sages of ancient India believed that improved technique is not the answer, but that transforming a solitary self-indulgent experience into something shared equally between both partners. The best love-making experience is understood in India to happen in a non-thinking, or 'mindless' state, where one's focus is completely on one's partner. Delaying orgasm is the most effective way a man can bring himself into the present. The classic Indian sex manual, the Kama Sutra, is actually an appraisal of female sexual response, showing ways to heighten desire and increase the loving connection with your partner. For the more that your sex life is little more than mutual masturbation, the more you want of it and the less satisfying it becomes. Making love to your chosen partner, however, and being 'in the moment' together is the most important element of a fulfilling sex life. If your husband is experiencing problems because of premature ejaculation or impotency, the best treatment is to use a combination of the herbs recommended for men, and working to eliminate stress. Meditation is very beneficial here, as is physical exercise. A diet that lowers toxins is also recommended for several weeks (light whole grains such as basmati rice and barley, pure water, steamed vegetables, fruit eaten by itself, and the avoidance of dairy products, meat and fish), followed by a low protein diet.

Pep up an Ailing Sex Life

To reintroduce the vitality of the sexual experience into your love life, try the following Ayurvedic technique which is known as 'passive intercourse' for at least a month. Unite with your partner and stay completely still, neither of you should move but should stay in this unified position, perhaps curled up in the spoons position, for at least 20 minutes and up to an hour if you can. This will increase the sense of intimacy you feel and remove sexual tension from the act of intercourse. It refocuses the emphasis on being together in a loving way and removes the need to reach a sexual high while you reacclimatize to each other. But once is not enough, you need to rediscover each other through this very intimate form of touching a couple of times to feel the real benefits, and then continue mutual passivity even if you feel sexual urges developing. Focus on each other and how lovely it would be to continue, and within a few weeks your desire should be rekindled.

Aphrodisiacs

Ayurveda has a lot to say about the use of aphrodisiacs, but it is important to understand their purpose. The Ayurvedic usage of the term aphrodisiac means the *health* of the sexual organs. They are given to rejuvenate the sexual organs and to help create happy children – not to create disproportionate desire where it is flagging or non-existent. In those cases it is better to abstain and wait until sexual energy returns of its own volition. However, the daily ingestion of certain plants and foods is believed to help increase

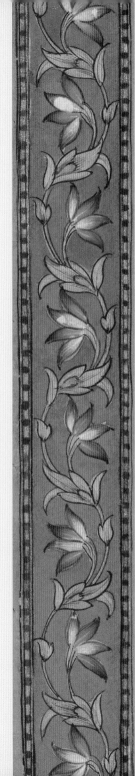

the vitality of the sperm and the egg. Aphrodisiacs are believed to increase the likelihood of a healthy child and increase the enjoyment of making love to your partner. The *Charaka Samhita*, an ancient Vedic text, points out with prosaic clarity that the best aphrodisiac of all is someone who loves you. Working to create a loving relationship in which you are attracted to such close proximity to your partner is a much better way of improving your sex life rather than relying on medicines and herbal preparations.

Compatibility and Your Type

Your type affects your physical, spiritual and emotional constitution, and therefore has an impact upon your personality and the sort of relationship you choose to create. Generally speaking, Air types are unpredictable, sometimes being submissive, but suddenly reasserting themselves. Earth types enjoy harmony and will go to immense lengths to achieve it, while Fire types are strong expressive characters who tend to wear the trousers. Like types tend to attract, and opposite types often complement one another - but how positive your relationship is depends on how balanced your own type is. Few people are truly composed of one type however, which makes for interesting, original and dynamic interactions as the different elements of two personalities meld and change. The following points shed some useful light:

Fire people are always drawn to a challenge, and if they can control their appetite for adventure, two Fire souls can enjoy an immensely rewarding and creatively stimulating relationship. They will feed each others sexual and artistic appetites and sparks will fly, positively and negatively. But if the couple have excess Fire in their blood they will end up locked in a duel, always tussling to be leader and engaging in a very draining and unhealthy game of control chess.

Earth types tend to be relaxed, contented, happy people. One reason is that they are naturally calm, but this can lead them to become rather lazy. Two Earth types together can enjoy an immensely satisfying and gentle union when they coax each other to eat well, get out and about, and share new experiences. But if they become too lazy, they can quite easily become couch potatoes who gradually go to seed and end up feeling rather resentful of the other's lack of drive.

Air types are drawn to balance and relaxation, but if they cannot find or create this backdrop to their relationship they can become rather frustrated and irritable. What has the potential to be a stimulating and nurturing relationship can tip the scales into a rather fractious union if they are not balanced when they meet.

Simple aphrodisiac approaches:

An active lifestyle – if you are sedentary, spend your whole time watching television and don't get regular exposure to fresh Air your 'prana' or sexual energy is likely to become dormant.

A healthy, light, vitamin-rich diet – eating masses of heavy rich food will stop your sexual energy being able to flow.

An active sex life – long-term abstinence and celibacy is not a healthy path to follow unless you have a naturally low sex drive.

Honey mixed in milk – warm the drink if you are a Fire type, otherwise Air and Earth types should drink it cold.

Making love at night – this will encourage your sexual energy to keep flowing during the day, rather than becoming depleted by having sex in the mornings.

Making love in the winter – the higher temperatures of the summer heats the body excessively leading to an increase in Fire energy and stamping out the influence of the Earth energy which controls the sexual fluids (NB This is probably less of an issue in the British climate, but might explain why you can feel less like sex on that expensive tropical holiday).

Aphrodisiac Herbs

The following herbs are all feted in Ayurvedic texts for their positive effects on the reproductive system (see also pages 68 to 73 on supplements). They are available in the UK and are safe and effective if taken correctly. Always follow the recommended dosage. Taking a large dose won't create a stronger effect, but could be dangerous. To gain benefits the herbs must be used long-term and only ever in the quantities suggested, these are not super-quick-fixes and taking more of them won't speed up the effects.

For Men:

Amla: One of the most famous Ayurvedic herbs, amla is renowned for its male rejuvenating properties. The fruit has the highest proportion of vitamin C to be found in nature – 20 times more than orange juice. Clinical studies show that it increases the red blood cell count and reduces cholesterol. It is the perfect daily health supplement. Dosage: 2 to 4 grams a day with meals.

Ashwagandha: In India this root of the winter cherry is a well known semen promoter and is also used to treat infertility and impotence in men. Clinical studies show that it has antibacterial, anti-inflammatory, and anti-tumour effects. It also helps to harmonize immune function, stabilize low blood pressure and regulate heartbeat. Dosage: 2 to 4 grams a day with milk or warm water.

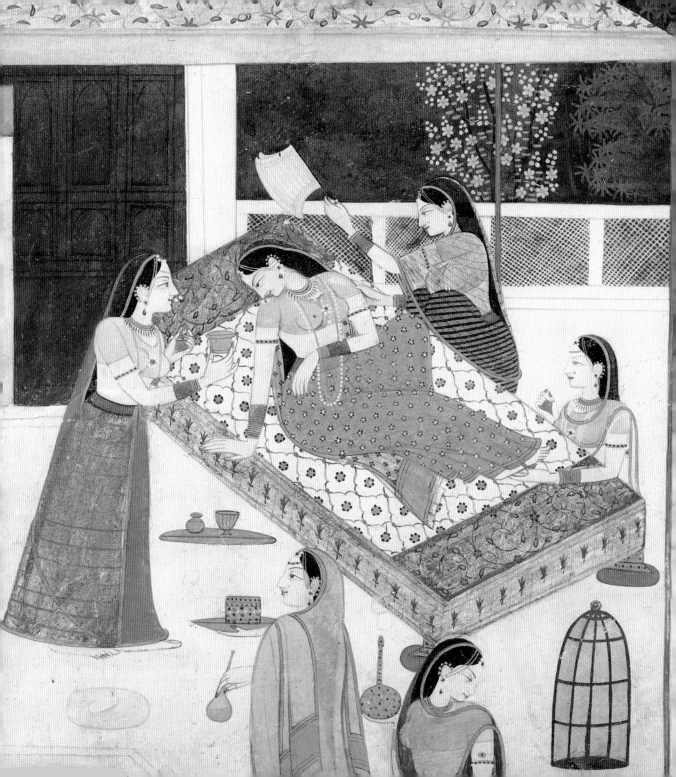

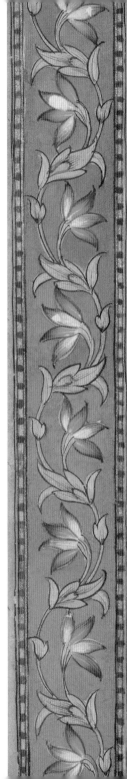

Guggulu: The gum from a tree related to myrrh, guggulu is used as the base for many Ayurvedic herbal preparations. It also reduces fat and toxins, is effective in treating arthritis, and is reputed to have aphrodisiac properties for men. Dosage: Two 450mg tablets with meals, three times a day.

Haritaki: Known as 'the King of Medicines' in Tibet, it is the mainstay of the Ayurvedic herbal tradition, is renowned as the best male aphrodisiac and is reputed to have extraordinary healing powers. Clinical studies have shown that it is effective against the herpes simplex virus, has antibacterial properties, increases the life of tissues and is even used to inhibit the HIV virus. Dosage: 2 to 5 grams per day.

For Women:

Kumari: Taken in a fresh gel format this is renowned for its female rejuvenating properties, but should be avoided during pregnancy. It is well known in the USA where it is often prescribed for disorders of the female reproductive system. You will need to take it daily for two menstrual cycles before observing results. Dosage: Two tablespoons of gel twice a day.

Shatavari: This form of asparagus is considered to be the most effective general tonic for women known to Ayurveda and is an excellent daily supplement for all women (unless they are obese when it should be avoided). It is the primary aphrodisiac for women (remember, this means for creating health in the sexual organs) and in Sanskrit means 'possesses a hundred husbands'! You need to use it regularly for a minimum of three menstrual cycles before seeing benefits. It is a phytooestrogen (a naturally occurring oestrogen) which aids a woman's long-term health, helping to prevent the incidence of breast cancer and osteoporosis without increasing the risk of uterine cancer like some synthetic hormones. For men it is believed to aid erectile tissue, especially when used in combination with ashwagandha. Dosage: 2 to 6 grams a day with meals.

Preparing to Conceive

Traditional Ayurvedic teaching believes strongly in the nature side of the nature/nurture debate. This long running philosophical, psychological and biological debate addresses whether our personalities are formed from our experience (the so-called 'tabula rasa' - or blank slate - approach) or whether our fundamental soul is determined at the moment of conception. Ayurveda inclines towards the latter. Because of this, there is much Ayurvedic teaching about preparing for the moment of conception, ensuring that both partners are in good health and able to produce the best quality sperm and egg possible.

Although doctors in the West tend not to issue advice on conception unless a couple are having difficulty in achieving a pregnancy, Ayurvedic doctors outline a thorough detoxification programme before conceiving. Strict Ayurvedic practitioners will therefore encourage a young couple to prepare for conception by undergoing application of oils, sweat therapy, laxative treatments and even therapeutic vomiting. The belief is that these approaches will help achieve the right balance of Air, Earth and Fire in the sperm and the egg.

A simple way of incorporating this belief into your life is to try the following advice for a month or so prior to conception: Women should introduce sesame into their diet, while men should increase their intake of milk and use ghee (clarified butter) in place of butter. Both of them should eat a healthy diet and avoid stress.

Ayurveda suggests that the perfect time to attempt to conceive is on the fourth day after the end of the last period. Ayurveda suggests that the couple should not make love for three days and the woman should avoid massage or any strenuous activity in order to 'still' the body in preparation. On the day of attempted conception the Ayurvedic texts suggest a woman should wear white and the man should wear fresh flowers in his buttonhole. The couple should focus on the quality and meaning of their relationship, concentrating on the strong feelings they have for one another and their desire to have a child. They should visualize a healthy baby, listen to uplifting music, take special care of their appearance and create a sense that this is a special day. Conception is believed to be more likely if the woman lies on her back (probably because the sperm is more likely to stay inside her for a while).

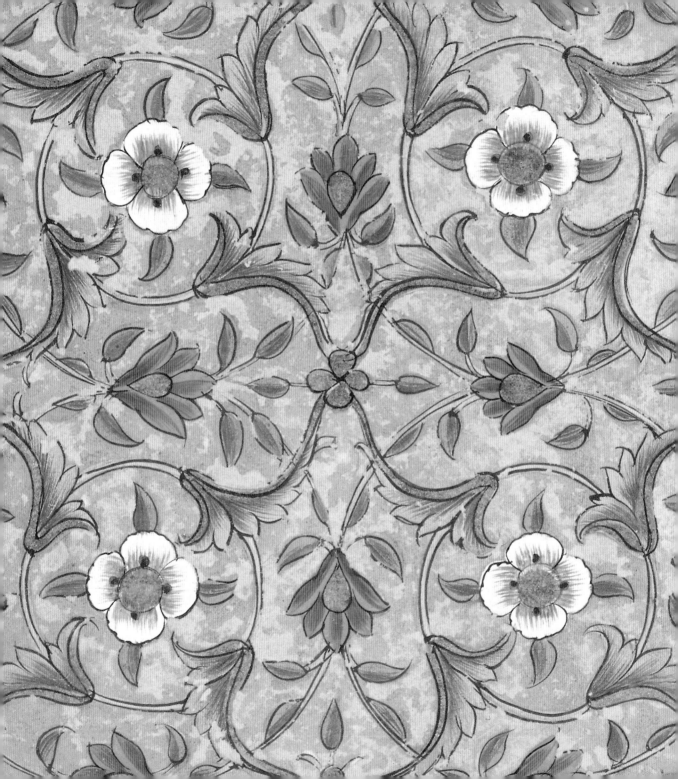

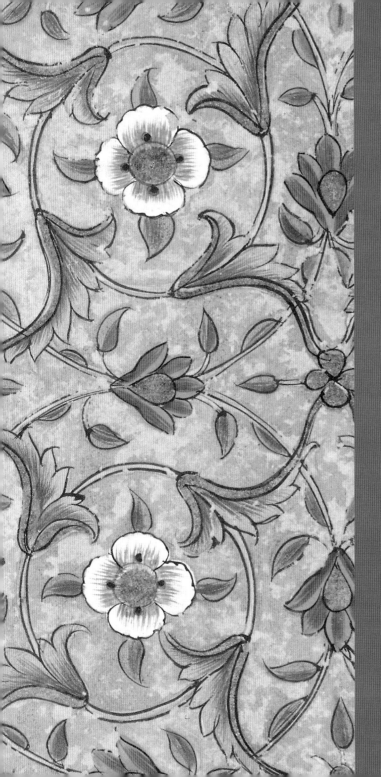

Balancing

Your Life Through Food

and Water

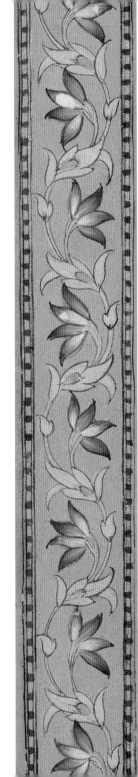

Ayurveda and Nutrition

Vedas: Food is life-force: life-force is food.

Hippocrates: Let food be your medicine and medicine your food.

Nutrition lies at the core of Ayurveda, so my heartfelt thanks goes out to Dr Jeannette Ewin for writing this section. She has transformed my Indian recipes, and translated Ayurvedic teachings, to offer delicious recipes and wonderful advice which will make you look and feel great.

This section explains how to prepare and enjoy food in the most beneficial way. I am a practical woman, and know that it is not easy to change everything in your life at once. Change must come in stages. For that reason, I have kept things as simple as possible. In the following pages you will read how to prepare and enjoy eating food. You will learn about the importance of water. You will find lists of foods that will help you balance your dosha. And, you will find a few recipes that can get you started on an amazing journey to better health.

All health programmes based on food choices agree that there is a strong connection between eating the wrong foods and illness. In Ayurveda, specific foods are used to balance – or correct – the physical, emotional and spiritual conditions that cause disease. This is totally unique to Ayurveda,

In Ayurveda nutrition is seen as being the

unlike concepts used in modern nutrition. However, many of the results are surprisingly similar.

For example, people dominated by Earth (kapha), tend to be slow in their movements, and to gain weight. They need food that is full of spices and herbs to satisfy their hunger, but at the same time they need foods low in fats. With time, foods chosen to reduce Earth will also result in weight loss. In a similar manner, in people dominated by Air (vata), there is a tendency to become anxious, tense, and to lose weight. Enjoying a diet based on Ayurvedic food provides a calming diet. By studying the food charts at the end of this section, you will see that many of these foods provide plenty of the B-complex vitamins needed for a healthy – and calm – central nervous system.

I have asked that the recipes included here be created in the style of traditional Western food choices. They reflect the teaching of many experts, some of whom have written the books listed under references, but when prepared correctly, will fit into your everyday style of enjoying food. Spicy mushroom crêpes, roasted potato snacks, and walnut bars are healthy Ayurvedic foods that suit our modern lifestyle.

Vegetarians may be surprised to see a few recipes incorporating some form of animal flesh: prawns, for example. These are included because not everyone can completely exclude meat from their diet, or are unable to meet their body's requirement for protein from plant sources. I recognize this, although I am a vegetarian, and eat no flesh. The majority of others who practice Ayurveda are also vegetarians and avoid all forms of flesh, including eggs, which some believe are living creatures 'in waiting'. However, the ancient teachings of Ayurveda did not totally exclude meat, but did stress that the animals from which this came should be treated with respect. This is the key: respect all living things, and do not eat as though food is something produced without the giving of life. Organic farming is the kindest way to produce the food we need for life.

Nutrition basics:

In Ayurveda, specific foods are used to balance – or correct – the physical, emotional and spiritual conditions that cause disease.

key to physical, spiritual and emotional wellbeing.

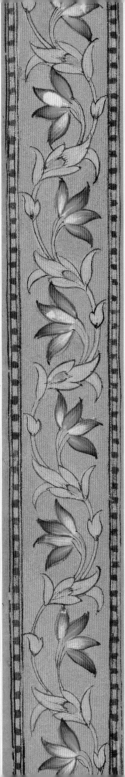

Love is the most important ingredient in Ayurvedic cooking. Your mood influences the flavour and appearance of everything you cook, and – it is believed – will be transferred to those who eat what you prepared. The Ayurvedic literature is full of stories about the passing of emotion from the person who prepares food to the person who eats it. One involves a man brought before a judge after committing a brutal crime. Witnesses speaking in his favour told how calm and kind he was; how unlike him it was to become violent. The judge studied the man for a long time, and then asked: 'Who prepared the last food you ate before committing this terrible crime?' A woman in the village, he was told; she was a good cook, but well known for beating her children and chasing her husband with a broom. 'Ah,' said the judge, 'then |you could not help yourself when you committed this crime. Her anger and violence entered you through the food she cooked, and affected your behaviour.' He was freed and told to eat what his wife prepared.

Ritual gives structure, and structure promotes feelings of calm. For this reason, I am recommending a series of little rituals and behaviours that will help you gain more from Ayurveda cooking.

When you prepare food

Respect the ingredients you use. These are part of life itself, and are to become part of you. Be aware of what you are handling: enjoy the colour, texture, and the aroma of the fruits, vegetables, nuts and seeds that go into your cooking bowl. And when you cook food, take time to observe how it changes during the process. Forget the microwave. If its only purpose is to speed up the process of getting dinner ready, it is robbing you of the *enjoyment* of seeing and smelling the food you are preparing.

If you are tense, take a few minutes to relax before going to the kitchen.

The kitchen reflects you and your moods more than any other room in the house. Place fresh flowers where they can be enjoyed as you cook.

Surround yourself with music that calms you.

Keep the kitchen clean. Wipe work surfaces. Remove your rings and jewellery before you touch any ingredients, and wash your hands well. Use your hands as you cook: it brings you closer to the ingredients.

When you eat

The environment should be cool, but the emotions should be warm and friendly.

Chew slowly: take time to taste your food, and feel it in your mouth.

Eat at a table: avoid sitting slouched in front of the television. Take no telephone calls during dinner, and side-step arguments. Slouching distorts the digestive system, promoting indigestion.

Even when the meal is very simple, place flowers on the table, and use candles at night. The flowers may be very simple, even a few wild blossoms will do. Candlelight softens the glare of artificial light.

Drinking water

This is a most important part of maintaining good health. Water cleans your internal body constantly. This is an unpleasant analogy, but you will understand my point: you use water in the toilet to carry away waste. You would certainly not want to continually use the same water. You want fresh water each time. It is like that in the body.

Some years ago I used to say that you should sip enough water throughout the day to equal $1\frac{1}{2}$ to two litres. People laughed. Now, it is popular to see people in the gym, or in the office, sipping bottled water.

Water is the internal sea in our bodies which contains the processes of life. It acts as a transport system, helps maintain normal body temperature, and acts as a catalyst in some chemical reactions.

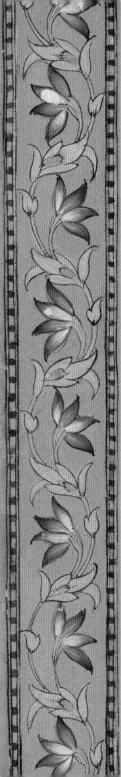

Rules for drinking water

Unless required as part of a healing treatment, distilled water should not be used for drinking, because it contains no minerals.

Drink minimal amounts of rainwater because it contains few minerals and may also contain toxic pollutants absorbed from the atmosphere as it falls.

Drink cool water to calm the body, but avoid ice water because it shocks the internal system. (The one exception is in the case of a high fever, when sipping ice water may help reduce fever.)

Drink filtered water or fresh spring water. Install a water filter in your kitchen so a fresh supply is always at hand for both cooking and drinking.

The value of adding fluorine to water is a hotly debated. It is not a mineral naturally found in the human body and its impact on the normal biological processes is unclear. Proponents claim it helps reduce the level of tooth decay. Opponents say it weakens the immune system and can cause genetic damage.

Tips

For a refreshing drink, add a slice of lemon or lime to a glass of cool water. This is an excellent alternative to soft drinks, and children should be encouraged to try it.

Unless you use a carbon filter every day, be sure to run water through it for at least a minute before using it for drinking water. They are an excellent means of removing impurities from drinking water; however they do not remove viruses or bacteria, which may remain in the filter and multiply.

When you buy bottled water, remember that natural mineral waters must come from recognized underground sources. As the mineral content varies from source to source, the taste of the water will also vary. Before bottling, the water may be filtered, and even carbonated; but no other substances can be added, including disinfectants.

Ceramic filters filter out bacteria as well as unwanted compounds in the water. Some remove certain minerals and soften the water.

Reverse osmosis filters are the most expensive and effective means of purifying water, and produce a product of medical quality. They eliminate bacteria and viruses, reduce levels of herbicides, pesticides and nitrates, and significantly clean the water of lead, mercury and other heavy metals.

If you drink bottled water, choose sparkling, because the carbon dioxide they contain inhibits the growth of bacteria. Still bottled water may contain bacteria because the water may be bottled and stored for more than a year, allowing organisms to multiply.

Do not use tap water for cooking. The chlorine used to control bacteria in public drinking water alters the taste of food and adds nothing to its nutritional value.

Eat foods that balance your doshas

Remember to listen to your body when you make food choices: on a hot summer day, you will not enjoy the same foods you want during winter.

Lists of foods that balance the three doshas:

	Increased	Decreased
Vata	pungent, bitter and astringent foods	sweet, sour and salty foods
Pitta	pungent, sour and salty foods	sweet, bitter and astringent foods
Kapha	sweet, sour, salty foods	pungent, bitter and astringent foods

There are six basic flavours in Ayurveda: sweet, sour, salty, pungent, bitter and astringent. Some of each flavour should be included in every meal. For foods associated with each flavour, follow this guide:

Sweet – carbohydrates, proteins, fat, nuts and meat.
Sour – citrus, tomatoes, cheese, salad dressing, aged and fermented food.
Salty – salt, soy sauce, tamari, vegetables seasoning blends.
Pungent – chilli pepper.
Bitter – green leafy vegetables, tea, coffee, pure chocolate.
Astringent – lentils, beans, tea.

Food combinations to be avoided

Milk and meat
Jaggery (unrefined cane sugar) and honey
Milk with citrus fruit, coconut, or leafy vegetables
Honey and ghee in equal portions
Lemon with milk, yoghurt, cucumbers or tomatoes (This does not hold when preparing paneer cheese.)
Eggs with milk, meat, yoghurt or cheese

1. Ghee

Makes about 225g/8oz/1 cup

There is no substitute for ghee or clarified butter. Do not use margarine or low-fat butter in the preparation of Ayruvedic foods.

clarified butter
250g/9oz/1 cup butter

1. Slowly melt the butter in a bain-marie, or small pan heated over boiling water. The butter fat will separate from the water and protein that form part of all butters.
2. Gently pour off the fat, leaving the watery residue behind, or place the pan in the refrigerator until the butter hardens.
3. Once solid, lift it from the dish and scrape off any residue that remains on the bottom of the butter.

A slightly more authentic flavour can be achieved by adding 1–2 whole cloves to the butter as it melts.

If you wish to reduce	Air	Fire	Earth
Eat	more	more	less

Ghee is highly acclaimed in Ayurvedic medicine for its healing properties, as it is believed to both purify and disinfect.

Ghee is a vital ingredient in Ayurvedic cooking, and can be purchased in Asian food stores and from some large supermarket chains. It has a distinctive flavour, will not burn when used in frying, and will keep unrefrigerated for months. In reality, it is clarified butter, but made from yoghurt, not milk. If you cannot buy ghee in your area, you can make your own clarified butter, although it will have a slightly different taste.

2. Cooked Indian tomato salsa

Makes about 200g/7oz/1¼ cups

4–5 ripe plum tomatoes

1 small red chilli, de-seeded (small chillies are fiery, so do not touch your face or eyes while working with them; wash your hands well after touching.)

1 tbsp red wine vinegar

2 cloves garlic, chopped

½ tsp ground black pepper seeds

½ tsp turmeric

½ tsp sea salt

black pepper from a few turns of a pepper mill

2 tbsp olive oil

1. Combine all the ingredients in a heavy pan and place over medium heat. Stir to help release the moisture from the tomatoes.
2. Reduce heat to low, and cook until thickened. Stir occasionally to prevent sticking.
3. Remove to a small container with a tight lid. Cool and refrigerate.

If you wish to reduce	Air	Fire	Earth
Eat	some	less	some

Excellent when served with cheese, or as a relish with rice and dhal.

3. Paneer

Makes about 100g/3 1/2 oz/1/2 cup, depending on the quality of the milk

There are many recipes for paneer, but here is one of the easiest. Note that it calls for whole milk. Nothing else will do.

1 litre /35fl oz/4 1/2 cups fresh whole milk
juice of 1/2 fresh lemon

1. Pour the milk into a large pan and place over medium heat. While stirring, bring the milk to the boil.
2. Reduce the heat to low and add the lemon juice. Continue stirring and cooking the mixture until large curds form. The fluid released from the curds – the whey – will have a yellowish colour.
3. Prepare to make the cheese by lining a colander with clean cheesecloth, and placing it over a larger vessel. Pour the curdled milk through the cheesecloth. Tie the ends of the cloth and suspend over the sink or a pan for at least 1 hour to drain off as much fluid as possible. (You can press the bag with your hands to speed up the process.) This soft cheese can be used in salads or spread in sandwiches.
4. For a firmer cheese, place the cheese – still in the cloth – in a bowl and weight down with a heavy object to continue extracting the whey. Leave in the refrigerator overnight if possible. When finished, remove the cheesecloth and refrigerate the cheese. Don't be surprised by the small amount of cheese produced from 1 litre/35fl oz/4 1/2 cups of milk.

Paneer is a fresh white cheese widely used in Ayurvedic cooking. It can be purchased in many Asian food stores, and in some major supermarket chains. If you cannot find a source in your area, you can make your own, or substitute similar cheese. Avoid products that have been salted (feta, for example) or have a rind. Processed cheeses are totally inappropriate in this style of cooking. Paneer is a good source of complete protein, but remember that it contains fat. As this recipe does not work with skimmed, or semi-skimmed, milk, you should find another source if you are Earth.

If you wish to reduce	Air	Fire	Earth
Eat	some	some	some

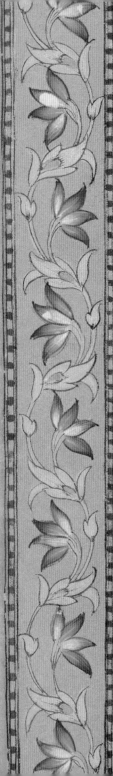

4. Rice

Use Basmati rice in your cooking. It is acceptable for balancing all three doshas. Basmati is a most attractive rice, with long white grains and the gentle aroma of flowers. To prepare, either follow the instructions on the package, or try the following method:

Serves 6

400g/14oz/2 cups long-grain rice
1 litre /35fl oz/4¹/₂ cups water

1. Wash the rice several times, cover with fresh water and allow to stand for at least 15 minutes.
2. Drain the rice and place in a heavy pan with a tight fitting lid. Add the water. Place the uncovered pan over a high heat and bring to the boil. Reduce the heat to a simmer and cook for 4–5 minutes. Cover the pan, remove from the heat and allow to stand for 20 minutes. Stir once during this time.
3. Leave the rice in the pan until you are ready to serve it. If there is unabsorbed water in the pan, return it to the heat and cook until the water is absorbed.

If you wish to reduce	Air	Fire	Earth
Eat	more	more	more

5. Buckwheat pan scones

For 10–12 scones

2 eggs

300ml/10fl oz/1⅓ cup Greek yoghurt

175g/6oz/1¼ cups buckwheat flour

½ tsp salt

½ tsp bicarbonate of soda (baking soda)

1 tsp cream of tartar

vegetable oil for cooking

1. In a large mixing bowl, whisk together the eggs and yoghurt.
2. Add flour and salt, and whisk until smooth.
3. Allow to 'rest' for at least 30 minutes at room temperature.
4. Just before cooking, add the bicarbonate of soda (baking soda) and cream of tartar to the flour mixture and blend well.
5. Coat the bottom of a heavy pan with a thin film of oil and place over medium heat. When the oil begins to 'swim', or move about on the surface of the pan, drop 2–3 spoonfuls of batter onto the oil. It will spread some, and begin to rise at once.
6. When bubbles in the scones break through the top, turn them and brown the other side. Cook until browned. Remove to a plate and cool.

These little cakes can be served at once, or refrigerated for another time. To reheat, drop into a toaster. A pleasing brown in' colour, they are attractive when served with green salad.

Enjoy: Freshly made, with a selection of roasted vegetables, toasted, then dotted with clarified butter, and topped with date syrup, or toasted, then heaped with sliced fresh strawberries and yoghurt.

Buckwheat is rich in rutin, which helps curb capillary fragility. Gluten-free, this much neglected grain is a good substitute for wheat.

If you wish to reduce	Air	Fire	Earth
Eat	more	some	less

6. Savoury crêpes

Makes 10–12 crêpes

150g/5^1/2oz/1 cup chickpea (gram) flour
^{1}/2 tsp salt
^{1}/2 tsp cumin
250ml/8fl oz/1 cup water
vegetable oil

1. Whisk the flour, salt, cumin and water together until they form a smooth batter. The consistency should be that of light/single cream. Leave standing for at least 15 minutes.
2. Drizzle a little oil into a hot crêpe pan, or non-stick frying pan. Pour a small ladleful of batter into the hot pan. Wait until it bubbles on top and is brown underneath. Turn, cook a few seconds longer, and then remove to a plate.
3. Stack crêpes as you work.

Crêpes can be used at once, stored (covered) in the refrigerator up to 48 hours, or wrapped and frozen for up to 1 month.

If you wish to reduce	Air	Fire	Earth
Eat	some	some	less

7. Roasted vegetables

Baking food adds more warming qualities to food than steaming or simmering, and greatly enhances flavours. It reduces moisture and concentrates the sweet, natural flavours of most foods, and is an *easy* way to prepare tasty vegetables. Remember, however, that the volume shrinks, making servings smaller.

Select three or four varieties of vegetables appropriate to balance your body (dosha). When you shop, choose only the firmest vegetables

Vegetables that roast well include Jerusalem artichokes, tomatoes, courgette (zucchini) and other summer squash, aubergine, fennel, asparagus, yams and sweet potatoes. (See recipe on page 151.) Sweetcorn should be wrapped in aluminium foil before roasting: use only freshly picked corn.

2/3 lb selection of vegetables

3 tbsp olive oil (the amount will vary with the number

and types of vegetables you are using.)

1 tsp salt

1 tsp finely ground black pepper

Preheat oven to 200°C/ 400°F/Gas 6.

1. Cut vegetables into pieces. Cut courgette (zucchini) and tomatoes into quarters. Peel and slice aubergines (eggplants) into pieces no more than $1^{1}/_{4}$ cm/$^{3}/_{4}$ inch thick. Peel Jerusalem artichokes and cut in half. Split fennel bulbs in half.

2. Place the oil, salt and pepper in the bottom of a large bowl. Add the prepared vegetables.

3. With clean hands, devoid of jewellery, mix the dressing and vegetables together, rubbing the oil over all the surfaces.

4. Place the vegetables close together on a non-stick baking tray. Bake for 20–30 minutes, or until browned and tender.

Vegetables are low in fat, contain valuable minerals and vitamins, and provide important phytochemicals, such as antioxidants, that help protect against certain forms of cancer and heart disease.

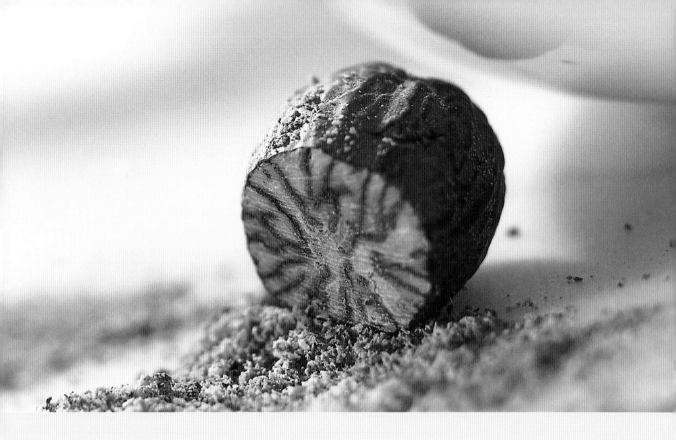

Note:

Aubergine (eggplant) should be sliced, placed on a non-stick baking tray, and lightly brushed on top with oil. Sprinkle with a little salt and black pepper.

    Tomatoes should be quartered, placed close together on a baking tray and drizzled with olive oil, and lightly sprinkled with salt and pepper.

    Asparagus should be rubbed in oil and seasoning, placed in a shallow baking pan, and baked until tender.

Roasted vegetables can be eaten on the day they are cooked, or stored in the refrigerator for future use. Trays of tomatoes, seasoned, roasted and dried in a slow oven, are delicious and make an excellent addition to salads, couscous, sandwiches and innumerable other dishes.

If you wish to reduce	Air	Fire	Earth
Eat vegetables listed for your dosha			

8. Spicy roasted sweet potatoes (A delicious snack food!)

Serves 6

olive oil

4 small sweet potatoes (peeled and washed)

2 tsp paprika

$1/2$ tsp chilli powder

salt

pepper

thyme sprig, to garnish

Preheat oven to 220°C/425°F/Gas 7

1. Pour enough olive oil into a large roasting pan to just cover bottom. Place in the oven 2–3 minutes or until hot.
2. Rinse and dry potatoes. Cut each one into eight wedges. Carefully spoon into hot oil, avoiding splashing.
3. Bake on top rack of the oven for 10 minutes, then turn the potatoes over and bake for 10 minutes more, until golden on the outside and cooked through.
4. Mix spices together. Using a slotted spoon, transfer potatoes to a serving dish. Sprinkle with spices, salt and pepper and stir well to coat evenly.
5. Bake for 20–25 minutes, or until tender when tested with a fork.
6. Serve hot, garnished with thyme.

If you wish to reduce	Air	Fire	Earth
Eat	more	some	less

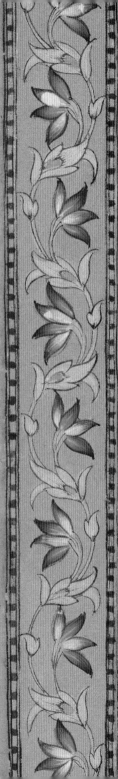

9. Red lentil dhal

Serves 4–6

250g/9oz/1 1/8 cup red lentils

100g/3 1/2oz/1 cup finely chopped onion

1 tsp sea salt

1 tsp freshly ground coriander (cilantro)

1 tsp ground cumin

1 tsp turmeric

1/2 tsp chilli powder

1 tsp dried tarragon

1. Pour the lentils into a large, heavy pan, cover with twice the volume of water and soak overnight.
2. The next day, drain, rinse, and cover with twice the volume of water.
3. Place the pan over a medium heat and bring to the boil. Lower the heat and simmer for 20 minutes, stirring occasionally.
4. Add the onion and salt. Turn up the heat and boil off the water, stirring as you do so. (Listen to the sound of the lentils as they cook. The sound of the bubbles will deepen as the mixture cooks. Cook, stirring constantly, until the bubbles are large, dry, and give a sighing, 'plopping' sound as they break. Cook off as much water as you dare before transferring the mixture to a heat-proof bowl.)
5. Add the spices and tarragon to the lentils and stir well.

The lentils are now ready to serve, or they may be covered and refrigerated overnight to use in a main course. (See page 164.)

If you wish to reduce	Air	Fire	Earth
Eat	more	some	more

10. Beverages

Use top quality ripe fruit in these recipes for the best taste. Make these drinks just before serving.

Pink delight

Serves I

¹/₄ ripe cantaloupe melon

115g/4 oz/⁴/₅ cup ripe strawberries

250ml/9fl oz/1 cup fresh pineapple juice

I tsp date syrup

1. Scoop the flesh from the melon.
2. Place all the ingredients in a blender and mix until smooth.
3. Pour and serve.

If you wish to reduce	Air	Fire	Earth
Eat	more	more	less

Sunrise

Serves I

I Sharon fruit

I ripe banana

200ml/7fl oz/³/₄ cup natural low-fat yoghurt

I tbsp orange juice

1. Remove the lid-like stem segment from the Sharon fruits and, using a small spoon, scoop the flesh out from the tough outer skin.
2. Place all the ingredients in a blender and mix until smooth.
3. Pour and serve.

If you wish to reduce	Air	Fire	Earth
Eat	more	some	less

Ayran

Serves 1

200ml/7fl oz/³⁄₄ cup natural low fat yoghurt
2 tbsp chopped fresh mint
few grains only of sea salt
250ml/9fl oz/1 cup cool sparkling water (still water can be used, but a slight effervescence is pleasant.)

1. Place the yoghurt, mint and salt in a blender and whizz until the pieces of mint are very small and the mixture has a slight green tone.
2. Add the water and whizz for only 1–2 seconds.
3. Serve at once.

This refreshing drink helps support a healthy digestive system.

If you wish to reduce	Air	Fire	Earth
Eat	more	less	less

11. Vegetable bouillon

Makes 750ml/25fl oz/3¼ cups

1 large sweet onion, thinly sliced

1 leek, chopped

2 celery stalks, chopped

3 carrots, chopped

2 tomatoes, chopped

2 bay leaves

3 tbsp chopped fresh flatleaf parsley

2 tbsp dried thyme

1 tbsp dried rosemary

salt, to taste

½ tsp black peppercorns

1 litre/35fl oz/4½ cups water

1. Combine all the ingredients in a large pan. Cover, bring to the boil, and simmer for 40 minutes.
2. To reduce, and strengthen the flavour, uncover and boil rapidly for 5 minutes or until stock (bouillon) is reduced to ¾ litre/25fl oz/3¼ cups.
3. Strain the stock (bouillon) into a large bowl and refrigerate.

If you wish to reduce	Air	Fire	Earth
Eat	more	some	more

12. Clear vegetable soup

Serves 4

750ml/25fl oz/3¹/₄ cups vegetable stock (bouillon)
2 carrots, thinly sliced
2 stalks celery, thinly sliced
55g/2oz/³/₄ cup finely diced button mushrooms
55g/2oz/1 cup broccoli florets
110g/4 oz/¹/₂cup frozen green peas
1 courgette (zucchini), cut into small, irregular chunks
salt and freshly ground black pepper to taste
fresh flatleaf parsley sprigs, to garnish

1. Warm the stock (bouillon) in a large pan. Add the vegetables, bring to the boil, cover and simmer for 5–6 minutes.

Using the tables at the back of this section, select the vegetables that best suit your requirements, and add these to the above recipe.

If you wish to reduce	Air	Fire	Earth
Eat	some	more	more

13. Parsnip and courgette soup

Serves 4

150g/5oz baby parsnips, cut in strips

400g/14oz courgette (zucchini), topped and tailed and cut in strips

1 tbsp vegetable oil

25g/1oz ghee or clarified butter

50g/2oz/$^{1}/_{2}$ cup chopped shallots

500ml/18fl oz/2$^{1}/_{4}$ cups vegetable stock (bouillon)

salt and freshly ground black pepper, to taste

sesame seeds or natural yoghurt, to garnish

Pre-heat the oven to 200°C/400°F/Gas 6.

1. Place the parsnips and courgette (zucchini) in a bowl. Add the oil and toss the vegetables in it to coat. Place the vegetables in a baking pan and roast until the parsnips are soft when tested with a fork.

2. Over medium heat, melt the ghee and sauté the shallots until they are translucent.

3. Place the cooked vegetables in a blender or processor; add the ghee with the shallots and salt and pepper, to taste. Add the vegetable stock (bouillon) and blend until smooth.

4. Pour into a heavy pan and heat, but do not boil. To garnish, serve sprinkled with sesame seeds or a dollop of yoghurt.

Tip: if you do not want to heat the oven, place 150ml/5fl oz/$^{2}/_{3}$ cup of stock (bouillon) in a heavy pan, cut the vegetables into thin slices, cover the pan with a tight lid, and cook over a medium heat, until the parsnips are tender. Continue as above. This does not give the rich flavour provided by roasting and is a lighter soup that is welcoming on a warm summer evening.

If you wish to reduce	Air	Fire	Earth
Eat	more	more	less

14. Carrot soup

Serves 6–8

Carrots improve liver function and strengthen the spleen and pancreas. They are a rich source of the carotenoids believed to help reduce risk from cancer.

25g/1oz ghee

500g/18oz/3 cups grated carrots (clean and run through a food processor)

500ml/18fl oz/2¼ cups vegetable stock (bouillon)

1 tsp turmeric

100ml/3½fl oz/½ cup apple juice concentrate

400ml/14 fl oz water

salt and pepper, to taste

toasted seeds or nuts, for topping

Tip: if you are not using organic carrots, peel them before cooking to remove any pesticide residue.

1. Heat the ghee in a large pan and sauté the carrots until they are soft.
2. Add the stock (bouillon) and cook for 10 minutes.
3. Remove from the heat and allow to cool.
4. Place in a food processor or blender and purée until smooth.
5. Return to the pan, add the turmeric, apple juice concentrate and water and heat until the mixture begins to simmer.
6. Adjust the seasoning, to taste.
7. Pour into soup plates. Sprinkle with toasted seeds or nuts before serving.

If you wish to reduce	Air	Fire	Earth
Eat	more	more	some

15. Roasted vegetable sandwiches

Serves 1 (an excellent lunch)

1 pitta bread, split

2 thin slices paneer cheese (or other fresh white cheese)

slices of roasted vegetables that balance your dosha. (See recipe on page 149.)

1. Place the cheese on one side of the split bread, and fill with strips of roasted vegetable. Cold: Wrap sandwich tightly in plastic film and allow to stand for at least 15 minutes to allow flavours to blend. Open, cut, and enjoy.

   OR

Warm: close the sandwich and wrap in aluminium foil. Place in a warm oven [170°C/325°F/Gas 3] for 15 minutes. Open and serve with a green salad for a delicious light lunch.

Vegetables contain most of the micronutrients needed for good health. Roasting them reduces their fluid content, but concentrates their nutrients and flavour.

If you wish to reduce	Air	Fire	Earth
Eat	more	more	less

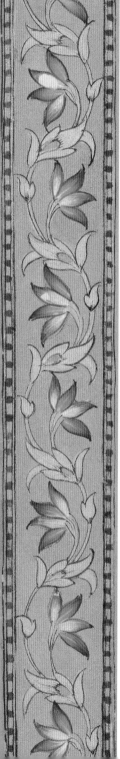

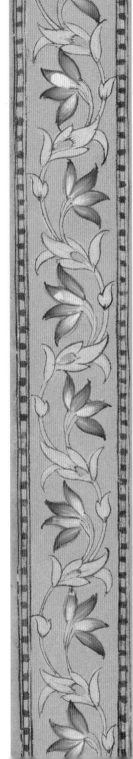

16. Buckwheat mini-pizzas

Serves 2

2 buckwheat pan scones (See recipe on page 147.)

4 slices paneer or other soft white cheese

2 tbsp cooked Indian tomato salsa (See recipe on page 144.)

fresh basil

Preheat grill (broiler).

1. Split the scones in half and place on a baking tray.
2. Layer the cheese on top and spread with salsa.
3. Place under hot grill (broiler), until the cheese begins to brown.
4. Remove and place on heated plates.
5. Garnish with torn pieces of fresh basil leaves.

This easy dish is a good source of vegetable nutrients, and contains useful amounts of protein.

If you wish to reduce	Air	Fire	Earth
Eat	some	some	some

17. Beet and egg salad

Serves 2

Dressing:

2 tbsp extra virgin olive oil

2 tbsp balsamic vinegar

salt and freshly ground black pepper, to taste

Salad:

60g/2¼oz/1 cup finely shredded iceberg lettuce

60g/2¼oz/⅓ cup cooked beetroot (beet), cut into thin sticks

2 hard-boiled free range eggs, peeled and quartered

4 handfuls greens, to serve

1. Mix together the oil and vinegar, and add the salt and pepper. Stir and set aside.
2. In a large bowl, combine the lettuce and beetroot (beet), add the salad dressing and toss, and divide between serving plates. Arrange the eggs on top of the vegetables.
3. Add 4 handfuls of greens – watercress, dandelion greens and alpha-alpha, for example. Toss lightly and serve.

If you wish to reduce	Air	Fire	Earth
Eat	more	some	more

Beetroot (beet) is acclaimed for its healing properties which are said to purify the blood, improve circulation and benefit the liver.

18. Couscous with goat's cheese and roasted vegetables

Serves 2

roasted vegetables (See page 149 for instructions.)
6 slices fresh goat's cheese
prepared couscous, according to packet instructions.

Dressing:

1 tbsp olive oil
2 tbsp lime juice
$^1/_2$ tsp sea salt
chopped fresh parsley, to serve

1. Warm the vegetables in a low oven [150°C/300°F/Gas 2], and set aside.
2. Place the cheese slices on a baking sheet and place under a hot grill, or 'blast' with a kitchen blowtorch until the edges brown.
3. Meanwhile, warm 2 dinner plates, and place a mound of couscous in the centre of each.
4. Arrange the roasted vegetables on top of the couscous, top with the cheese, and sprinkle with the dressing.
5. Sprinkle with chopped, fresh parsley. Serve at once.

If you wish to reduce	Air	Fire	Earth
Eat	more	some	less

19. Shiitake mushrooms *en crêpe*

Serves 2

150g/5oz/1 ¼ cups shiitake mushrooms, finely sliced

150g/5oz/1 ¼ cups button mushrooms, finely sliced

2 tbsp ghee or clarified butter

4 shallots, peeled and finely sliced

½ tsp sea salt

4 tsp cooked Indian tomato salsa (See recipe on page 144.)

4 crêpes (See recipe on page 148.)

fresh coriander (cilantro)

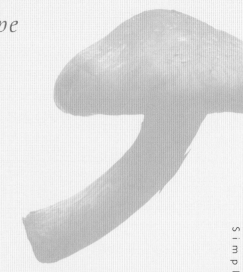

1. Prepare the mushrooms. Do not wash, simply brush or wipe away any bits of debris. Remove stems and slice.
2. Place ghee in a heavy skittle, or wok, and place over medium heat; when it begins to sizzle, add the shallots. Stir and cook until they begin to brown.
3. Add the mushrooms, salt and salsa, and cook until the mushrooms are limp.
4. To heat the crêpes, place on a warmed plate. The warming process should be gentle, as you do not want the crêpes to dry out or tear.
5. One by one, place the crêpes on serving plates and fill with half the mushroom mixture. Serve warm with a green salad.

Shiitake is one form of mushroom believed to help reduce the risk of solid cancers. They are said to be a natural source of interferon, which appears to enhance the immune response against viral diseases and cancer.

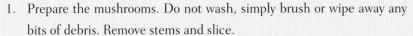

If you wish to reduce	Air	Fire	Earth
Eat	some	some	less

20. Red lentil patties with roasted vegetables

Lentils are an excellent source of iron, protein and B vitamins. To maximize the absorption of these nutrients, at the same meal, enjoy with foods rich in vitamin C. Roasted tomatoes are a good choice.

(See page 152 for instructions for cooking the lentils.)

(See page 149 for instructions for cooking the roasted vegetables.)

ghee, or clarified butter

chickpea (gram) flour

Making the patties:

1. Place about 2 tbsp of ghee in a heavy pan over medium heat and wait until it begins to bubble.

2. Take dessertspoon-size lumps of cold red lentil dhal from its container and, using your hands, form each into an elongated patty. The mixture should be firm.

3. After sufficient patties are shaped, dust your hands with gram flour. Drench each patty in the chickpea (gram) flour, encouraging a skin, or crust to form.

4. One by one, lower the patties into the heated ghee and cook over medium heat until a nudge at the edge shows the crust turning brown. When you are sure a good crust has formed, turn the patty and repeat the process on the opposite side. You may want to add a little more ghee to the pan as these cook, allowing small pieces to melt and slide under the cooking dhal.

5. Arrange warm roasted vegetables around the lentil patties. Serve with yoghurt or spicy mango chutney.

If you wish to reduce	Air	Fire	Earth
Eat	more	some	less

21. Sweet and sour prawns

Serves 2

2 tsp hot chilli sauce

2 tbsp date syrup

1 tbsp cider vinegar

1 tbsp tomato purée (paste)

2 garlic cloves, crushed

225g/8oz/2 cups king prawns (shrimp) (5–6 per person). (If you are using frozen, use weight when thawed.)

2 tbsp vegetable oil

5–6 slices fresh ginger, shredded (use the most tender you can find)

1. In a large bowl, combine the chilli sauce, date syrup, cider vinegar, tomato puree (paste), and garlic. Stir to blend and add the prawns (shrimp). Stir again to coat prawns (shrimp) and allow to stand for 5 minutes.
2. Heat the oil in a wok, or heavy frying pan. Add the ginger and fry until it begins to brown.
3. Add the marinated prawns (shrimp) to the oil. Stir and fry until pink and cooked through. Do not allow the marinade to burn.
4. Remove from the heat at once. Place prawns (shrimp) on a bed of basmati rice.
5. Make a sauce by replacing the wok over the heat, and adding 1 tbsp water. Stir to combine the essence of the marinade, and pour over prawns (shrimp).

If you wish to reduce	Air	Fire	Earth
Eat	more	less	more

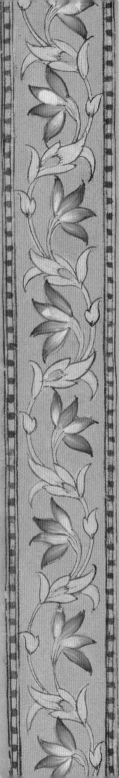

22. Figs with paneer cheese

Serves 2

4 ripe figs
225g/8oz/1 cup freshly made paneer cheese (See recipe on page 145.)

Dressing:

3 tbsp grape juice concentrate
1/4 tsp sea salt
zest of 1 lemon (organic)

1. Divide the paneer and place in the centre of two plates.
2. Quarter the figs and arrange around the cheese.
3. Blend the ingredients for the dressing and drizzle over the cheese.

(A sprinkle of toasted sunflower seeds over the salad adds texture and nutrients.)

If you wish to reduce	Air	Fire	Earth
Eat	more	some	less

Fresh fruit is an ideal addition to any meal. Based on the foods that suit your dosha, select fruit that will pep up the flavour of a salad, or make a pleasing and light end to a meal.

23. Apple Crystal

Serves 6

500ml/18fl oz/2 cups concentrated apple juice

250ml/9fl oz/1 cup water

125ml/4fl oz/¹/2 cup freshly squeezed orange juice

145g/¹/2oz/¹/8 cup agar-agar (vegetarian gelatine)

¹/2 tsp ground cloves

¹/2 tsp cinnamon

¹/2 tsp freshly ground nutmeg

2 large or 3 medium-size, ripe bananas

Cinnamon, cloves and nutmeg contain natural antibacterial and antiviral compounds.

1. Combine fluid ingredients in a heavy pan and add agar-agar. Allow to soak for 10–15 minutes.
2. Bring the mixture to the boil.
3. Reduce heat, wipe down all agar-agar from the sides of the pan with a spatula, and simmer for 3–5 minutes, or until pieces of agar-agar are no longer visible.
4. Add spices, then stir and remove from the heat.
5. Allow the mixture to cool for 30 minutes, then stir in fruit. Pour into serving bowl and cool in refrigerator until set.

If you wish to reduce	Air	Fire	Earth
Eat	more	some	more

Serve with Greek yoghurt. Earth should delete bananas and sprinkle with toasted sesame seeds instead.

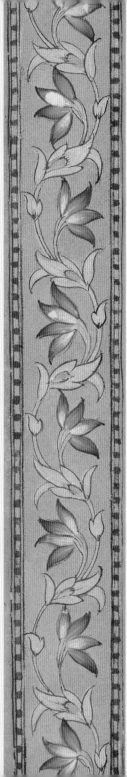

24. Date and almond slices

Serves 6–8

250ml/8fl oz/1 cup water

25g/1oz¹/₄ cup agar-agar (vegetarian gelatine)

250ml/8fl oz/1 cup date syrup concentrate

1 x 425g/14 oz can coconut milk

250g/9oz/3 cups ground almonds

1. Pour the water into a large pan and sprinkle agar-agar over the surface. The flakes are fine and will float on the water. Stir the mixture until all the flakes are wet, then allow to stand for 30 minutes.
2. Add the date syrup, stir and allow to stand for another 30 minutes.
3. Place the pan over a low heat and bring to the simmer. Stir and cook until the agar-agar is completely dissolved. (You can no longer see pieces on the back of a spoon.)
4. Add coconut milk and stir until completely blended.
5. Remove from the heat and cool for 1 hour.
6. Stir in the almonds and pour into a 900g/2lb loaf tin (pan).
7. Cover with clingfilm (plastic wrap) and place in the refrigerator until the mixture is set.
8. Dip the tin in hot water then invert the loaf onto a serving plate.
9. Cut into 1cm/¹/₂ inch slices. Arrange two slices on each dessert plate.

If you wish to reduce	Air	Fire	Earth
Eat	more	some	less

Air and Fire can top with yoghurt. Earth can top with sesame seeds.

25. Walnut angels

Makes 12–16 pieces

Pre-heat oven to 200°C/400°F/Gas 6
Grease a non-stick baking pan 23 × 30cm (9 inches × 12 inches) with ghee
or clarified butter

2 egg whites
¹/₂ tsp salt
110g/4 oz/¹/₂ cup jaggery (ground or powdered)
110g/4 oz/3 cups rice flour
110 g/4 oz/³/₄ cup corn flour (cornstarch)
2 tsp baking soda
110g/4 oz/⁴/₅ cup dates, finely chopped
110g/4 oz/1 cup walnuts, finely chopped

1. Whip the egg whites and salt until they form soft peaks.
2. Slowly add the jaggery, whipping constantly.
3. Sift the rice and corn flour (cornstarch) together with the baking soda.
4. Fold the flour mixture into the beaten egg whites.
5. Stir the dates and nuts into the mixture.
6. Spread over the greased pan and bake for 20–25 minutes.
7. Remove from the oven and score the cake to indicate where slices will
   be made.
8. Cool. Cut along the scored lines and remove from the baking pan.

If you wish to reduce	Air	Fire	Earth
Eat	more	some	less

Walnuts are rich in B vitamins that help control stress, and vitamin E and essential fatty acids that strengthen the heart. They are a good source of minerals and protein for vegetarians.

Enjoying foods to balance Air

Vegetables

Enjoy!	Enjoy Limited Amounts	Enjoy Small Portions
Beetroot (beet)	Asparagus	Artichokes
Carrots	Aubergines	Bean sprouts
Chilli peppers	Cauliflower	Beans (green)
Coriander (cilantro)	Celery	Broccoli
Courgette (zucchini)	Cucumber	Brussels sprouts
Fennel	Onions – cooked	Cabbage
Jerusalem artichokes	Spinach	Lettuce
Mustard greens		Mushrooms
Okra		Onions – raw
Parsley		Peas – green
Radishes		Potatoes
Seaweed		Squash – acorn
Sweet potatoes		Squash – winter
		Sweetcorn
		Sweet peppers
		(box)
		Tomatoes
		Turnips

Fruits

Enjoy!	Enjoy Limited Amounts	Enjoy Small Portions
Avocados	Apples	Cranberries
Blueberries	Apricots	Lemon/Orange zest
Cherries	Bananas	Melon
Dates	Oranges	Raisins/Currants
Figs	Peaches	/Sultanas
Grapefruit	Pears	
Grapes	Plums	
Lemons	Pomegranates	
Limes	Tangerines	
Mangoes		
Nectarines		
Papayas		
Pineapples		
Prunes		
Raspberries		
Blackberries		
Strawberries		

Pulses

Enjoy!	Enjoy Limited Amounts	Enjoy Small Portions
Mung (moong) beans	Aduki beans	Black gram
	Chickpeas (garbanzo beans)	Broad beans
	Kidney beans	Lentils
	Butter beans (lima beans)	Borlotti beans (pinto beans)
	Tofu	Soya beans
		Split peas

Grains

Enjoy!	Enjoy Limited Amounts	Enjoy Small Portions
Oats	Barley	Couscous
Basmati rice	Buckwheat	Muesli – dried grains
Brown rice	Corn	Rye
Spelt	Millet	White flour
Wholemeal flour	Quinoa	
	Refined white rice	

Dairy

Enjoy!	Enjoy Limited Amounts	Enjoy Small Portions
Butter	Cheese	Ice cream
Buttermilk	Paneer	
Cottage cheese		
Cream		
Ghee		
Milk		
Soured cream		
Yoghurt		

Nuts and Seeds

Enjoy!	Enjoy Limited Amounts	Enjoy Small Portions
Almonds	Coconut	Lotus seeds
Brazil nuts	Pumpkin seeds	Peanuts
Cashews	Sunflower seeds	
Hazelnuts		
Macadamia nuts		
Mustard seeds		
Pecans		
Pine nuts		
Pistachios		
Sesame seeds		
Walnuts		

Herbs and Spices

Enjoy!	Enjoy Limited Amounts	Enjoy Small Portions
Allspice	Black pepper	Anise
Asafoetida	Catnip	
Basil	Cayenne pepper	
Bay leaves	Dill	
Caraway	Horseradish	
Cardamom	Lemon verbena	
Camomile	Lemongrass	
Cinnamon	Mint	
Cloves	Mustard	
Coriander (cilantro)	Paprika	
Cumin	Peppermint	
Fennel	Spearmint	
Fenugreek	Turmeric	
Garlic		
Ginger		
Mixed Italian seasoning		
Marjoram		
Nutmeg		
Poppy seeds		
Rosemary		
Sage		
Star anise		
Tarragon		
Thyme		

Oils

Enjoy – Ghee, olive oil, most other oils

Use sparing amounts – Flaxseed

Sweeteners

Enjoy – Barley malt, fruit juice concentrate, raw honey, jaggery, molasses, rice syrup

Use sparing amounts – Maple syrup and white sugar

Animal Protein

(Always respect the animals from which these foods come.)

In small portions – Beef, chicken and turkey (white meat), duck, eggs, freshwater fish, shrimp

Enjoying foods to balance Fire

Vegetables

Enjoy!	Enjoy Limited Amounts	Enjoy Small Portions
Artichokes	Aubergines	Chilli peppers
Asparagus	Beetroot (beet)	Fennel
Bean sprouts	Carrots	Mustard greens
Beans (green)	Onions, cooked	Onions, raw
Broccoli	Parsley	
Brussels sprouts	Potatoes	
Cabbage	Radishes	
Cauliflower	Seaweed	
Celery	Spinach	
Coriander (cilantro)	Squash – acorn	
Courgette (zucchini)	Squash – winter	
Cucumbers	Sweetcorn	
Jerusalem artichokes	Sweet peppers (box)	
Lettuce	Sweet potatoes	
Mushrooms	Tomatoes	
Okra	Turnips/Swedes	
Peas – green		
Mange-tout (snow peas)		

Fruits

Enjoy!	Enjoy Limited Amounts	Enjoy Small Portions
Apples	Avocados	Apricots
Blueberries	Grapefruit	Bananas
Cranberries	Mangoes	Cherries
Dates	Nectarines	Lemons
Figs	Oranges	Limes
Grapes	Papayas	Peaches
Lemon/Orange zest	Plums	Tangerines
Pears	Raisins/Currants /Sultanas	Melons
Pineapples	Raspberries	
Prunes	Blackberries	
Pomegranates		
Strawberries		

Pulses

Enjoy!	Enjoy Limited Amounts	Enjoy Small Portions
Aduki beans	Chickpeas	
Black gram	(garbanzo beans)	
Broad beans	Kidney beans	
(fava beans)	Lentils	
Butter beans	Borlotti beans	
(lima beans)	(pinto beans)	
Mung (moong)	Soya beans	
beans	Split peas	
Tofu		

Nuts and Seeds

Enjoy!	Enjoy Limited Amounts	Enjoy Small Portions
Coconut	Pine nuts	Almonds
Lotus seeds	Pumpkin seeds	Brazil nuts
Sunflower seeds	Sesame seeds	Cashews
		Hazelnuts
		Macadamia nuts
		Mustard seeds
		Peanuts
		Pecans
		Pistachios
		Walnuts

Dairy

Enjoy!	Enjoy Limited Amounts	Enjoy Small Portions
Butter	Cheese	Buttermilk
Cottage cheese	Paneer cheese	Ice cream
Cream		Soured cream
Ghee		Yoghurt
Milk		

Grains

Enjoy!	Enjoy Limited Amounts	Enjoy Small Portions
Barley	Buckwheat	White flour
Couscous	Corn	
Oats	Millet	
Rice – basmati	Muesli – dried grain	
Spelt (coarse	Quinoa	
European wheat)	Rice – brown	
Wholemeal flour	Rice – refined, white	
	Rye	

Herbs and Spices

Enjoy!	Enjoy Limited Amounts	Enjoy Small Portions
Camomile	Basil	Allspice
Coriander	Caraway	Anise
(cilantro)	Cardamom	Asafoetida
Fennel	Catnip	Bay leaves
	Cinnamon	Black pepper
	Cloves	Calamus
	Cumin	Cayenne pepper
	Dill	Fenugreek
	Lemon verbena	Garlic
	Lemon grass	Ginger
	Mint	Horseradish
	Nutmeg	Hyssop
	Paprika	Italian seasoning
	Peppermint	Marjoram
	Rosemary	Mustard
	Saffron	Oregano
	Spearmint	Poppy seeds
	Turmeric	Star anise
		Tarragon
		Thyme

Oils

Enjoy – Canola (rapeseed) oil, ghee, olive oil, flaxseed oil, walnut oil

Use sparing amounts of – Avocado oil, coconut oil

Sweeteners

Enjoy – Barley malt, fruit juice concentrate, maple syrup, rice syrup

Use Limited Amounts of – Honey, jaggery (unrefined cane sugar), molasses, white sugar

Animal Protein

(Always respect the animals from which these foods come.)

In small portions – Chicken or turkey (white meat), egg white, freshwater fish, rabbit, prawn (shrimp)

Enjoying foods to balance Earth

Vegetables

Enjoy!	Enjoy Limited Amounts	Enjoy Small Portions
Asparagus	Artichokes	Cucumbers
Bean sprouts	Aubergines	Jerusalem artichokes
Beans (green)	Cauliflower	Onions, raw
Beetroot (beet)	Okra	Sweet potatoes
Broccoli	Parsley	Winter squash
Brussels sprouts	Potatoes	
Cabbage	Seaweed	
Carrots	Spinach	
Celery	Summer squash	
Chilli peppers	Sweetcorn	
Coriander (cilantro)	Sweet peppers (box)	
Courgette (zucchini)	Tomatoes	
Fennel		
Lettuce		
Mushrooms		
Mustard greens		
Onions, cooked		
Peas – green		
Mangetouts (snowpeas)		
Radishes		
Turnip/Swedes		

Fruits

Enjoy!	Enjoy Limited Amounts	Enjoy Small Portions
Apples	Apricots	Avocados
Cranberries	Papayas	Bananas
Grapefruit	Pears	Blueberries
Lemon/Orange zest	Prunes	Cherries
Raisins/Currants/	Pomegranates	Dates
Sultanas	Tangerines	Figs
		Grapes
		Lemons
		Limes
		Mangoes
		Melons
		Nectarines
		Oranges
		Peaches
		Pineapples
		Plums
		Raspberries
		Blackberries
		Strawberries

Dairy

Enjoy!	Enjoy Limited Amounts	Enjoy Small Portions
	Buttermilk	Butter
	Ghee	Cheese
	Paneer cheese	Cottage cheese
		Cream
		Ice cream
		Milk
		Soured cream
		Yoghurt

Nuts and Seeds

Enjoy!	Enjoy Limited Amounts	Enjoy Small Portions
Mustard seeds	Coconut	Almonds
	Peanuts	Brazil nuts
	Pumpkin seeds	Cashews
	Sesame seeds	Hazelnuts
	Sunflower seeds	Lotus seeds
		Macadamia nuts
		Pecans
		Pine nuts
		Pistachios
		Walnuts

Pulses

Enjoy!	Enjoy Limited Amounts	Enjoy Small Portions
Aduki beans	Black gram	Chickpeas
Broad beans	Kidney beans	(garbanzo beans)
Soya beans	Mung (moong)	
Lentils	beans	
Butter beans	Borlotti beans	
(lima beans)	(pinto beans)	
	Tofu	
	Split peas	

Grains

Enjoy!	Enjoy Limited Amounts	Enjoy Small Portions
Barley	Buckwheat	Couscous
Muesli – dried grains	Corn	Oats
Quinoa	Millet	Rice – brown
	Rice – basmati	Rice – refined, white
	Rye	White flour
	Spelt	Wholemeal flour

Herbs and Spices

Enjoy!	Enjoy Limited Amounts	Enjoy Small Portions	Enjoy!	Enjoy Limited Amounts	Enjoy Small Portions
Allspice	Catnip		Star anise		
Anise	Dill		Tarragon		
Asafoetida	Fennel		Thyme		
Basil	Lemon verbena		Turmeric		
Bay leaves	Lemon grass				
Black pepper	Mint				
Caraway	Nutmeg				
Cardamom	Paprika				
Cayenne pepper	Peppermint				
Camomile	Saffron				
Cinnamon	Spearmint				
Cloves					
Coriander (cilantro)					
Cumin					
Fenugreek					
Garlic					
Ginger					
Horseradish					
Hyssop					
Italian seasoning					
Marjoram					
Mustard					
Oregano					
Poppy seeds					
Rosemary					
Sage					

Oils

Enjoy – Almond oil, corn oil, ghee, Canola oil (rapeseed oil), sunflower seed oil

Use sparing amounts of – Soy, safflower oil, walnut oil

Sweeteners

Enjoy – Fruit juice concentrates, raw honey, concentrated date syrup

Use sparing amounts of – Barley malt syrup, fructose, jaggery (unrefined cane sugar), maple syrup, molasses, rice sugar, white sugar

Animal Protein

(Always respect the animals from which these foods come.)

In small portions – Chicken or turkey (dark meat), eggs, rabbit

Resources

Bharti Vyas' own range of Ayurvedic preparations was launched in January 2000. For mail order details call 020 7486 7167. Her London clinic offers a range of treatments inspired by the principles of Ayurveda, including Ayurvedic massage and rejuvenation treatments. The clinic also boasts a full-time Ayurvedic doctor among the therapy staff who has helped devise and supervises the treatments.

Where to find Ayurvedic ingredients and supplements

Local Indian supermarkets will stock many of the oils and herbs described, along with ghee and supplements.

Solgar Gold Label vitamins and Ayurvedic supplements (Ashwagandha, turmeric and Boswellin) are available from independent health food stores, to find the stockist nearest to you call 01442 890355. www.solgar.com

The Indian Food Centre (020 8888 1927) sells ingredients as well as Ayurvedic beauty preparations. 70 Turnpike Lane, Hornsey, London N8 OPR.

The Nutri Centre, 7 Park Crescent, London W1N 3HE. Tel: 020 7436 5122.

Himalaya USA sells Ayurvedic products and ingredients, 6950 Portwest Drive, Ste. 170, Houston TX 77024. Tel: 1800 869 4640.

The Himalayan Drug Company, c/o Vedic Medical Hall, 6 Chiltern Street, London W1M 1PAO. Tel: 020 7935 0028.

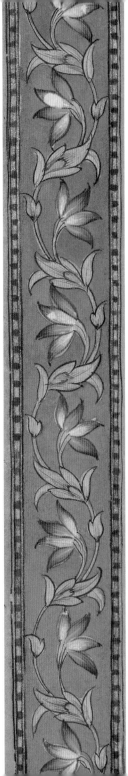

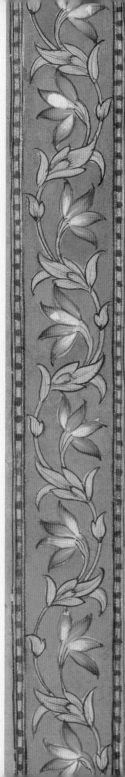

The Ayurvedic Trading Company Ltd, 10 St John's Square, Glastonbury, BA6 9LT, offers a practitioner prescription service, books and a full range of Ayurvedic herbs, both medicinal and culinary. Available by mail order on telephone: 01458 833382.

Where to go on Ayurvedic retreat

The Tyringham Naturopathic Clinic, Newport Pagnell, Milton Keynes, Buckinghamshire, MK16 9ER (01908 610450) is a registered non-profit making charity dedicated to providing the best of integrated health care in peaceful surroundings, including Ayurvedic options for treatment and lifestyle management. The clinic is based in a gracious Georgian villa with views across open countryside. The clinic philosophy is a belief that they do not help patients fight illness so much as discover wellness. Tyringham's senior consultant holds weekly consultations to prescribe a range of Ayurvedic herbs for internal ayurvedic treatment. These include tripala and trikatu for digestive problems, neem and mangista for skin problems, and Rumalaya tablets and creams for arthritic conditions. As well as a full range of other holistic therapies, Tyringham also offers external Ayurvedic treatments using dried herbs and hot oils. These are available one or two evenings a week.

 The Practice, The Manor House, Kings Norton, Leicestershire LE7 9BA (0116 259 6633) specializes in Ayurvedic retreats of varying duration from one to seven days, and only between one and four people at any one time stay at the centre where food eaten is often grown in the organic garden. Highlights include a five day full-on Panchakarma cleansing treatment experience, as well as a two-day quick fix, in a 17th century manor house set in a nine acre estate with fields, an organic garden and a farm. There are sessions and treatment sessions in holistic therapies including transformational breathing, yoga, subtle body healing, Tai Chi, Indian head massage and Ayurvedic lifestyle. Ayurvedic treatments are customized with the use of specified oils, herbs and aromas chosen to provide optimal balance and nourishment for mind/body constitution. An Ayurvedic doctor is able to ensure a complete and personalized diagnosis. Training courses are also available.

Ayurvedic Medical Clinics

These are the clinics to contact if you would like to refer an existing medical problem to a qualified Ayurvedic doctor:

Ayurveda at The Hale Clinic, 7 Park Crescent, London W1N 3HE. Tel: 020 7631 0156.

Ayurvedic Clinic, 322a St Albans Road, Watford, WD2 5PQ. Tel: 01923 246010.

Highfield Clinic, Highfield Lane, St Albans, Herts AL4 0RJ. Tel: 01442 66880.

Milton Keynes Ayurvedic Clinic, 17 Bromham Mill, Gifferd Park, Milton Keynes, Bucks, MK14 5QP. Tel: 01908 604 666.

Herbal Holiday Resorts (pvt) Ltd, 215/22/Nawala Road, Nugegoda, Sri Lanka. Tel 00 94 1 811 422.

Kappad Beach Resort, Kozhikode, Kerala, India. Tel: 00 91 496 683 760 www.kappadbeachresort.com

Kapl Ayurgram, Whitefield, Banglore, Kanataka, India. Tel: 00 91 080 5591 825

The Taj Malabar, Cochin, Kerala. Tel: 00 91 484 666 811.

Ayurvedic Beauty and Health Clinics

Contact these clinics if you would like to benefit from some of the cleansing, health and beauty regimes that Ayurveda has to offer:

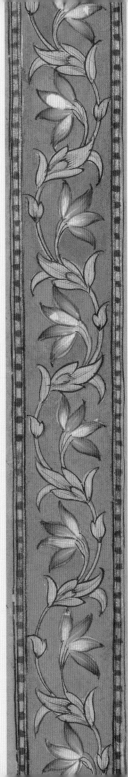

The Green Room offers treatments including the Ayurveda Experience. There are 10 London clinics, call 020 7937 6595 to find locations.

Maharishi Ayur-Veda Health Centre, 21 Clouston Street Glasgow G20 8QR. Tel: 0141 946 4663.

Tyringham and The Practice, both mentioned in the retreat section, also offer single sessions or day long Ayurvedic health and beauty experiences. Call for details.

Organizations

The Ayurvedic Medical Association (UK), the professional body of Ayurvedic physicians c/o The Hale Clinic, 7 Park Crescent, London W1N 3HE. Tel: 020 7631 0156.

Ayurvedic Company of Great Britain, 50 Penywern Road, London SW5 9SX. Tel: 020 7370 2255.

Practical Ayurveda (020 8866 5944) offers courses, both group or one-to-one, residential or single day, teaching the principles of Ayurveda for lifestyle management.

California College of Ayurveda, 117A East Main Street, Grass Valley, CA 95945. www.ayurvedacollege.com.

Meditation & Yoga

Transcendental Meditation Centre, 4 West Newington Place, Edinburgh, EH9 1QT. Tel: 0131 668 1649.

VinYoga Britain, PO Box 158, Bath BA1 2YG, maintains the UK register of yoga practitioners trained in small groups and one-to-one teaching and therapy.

The Yoga for Health Foundation, Ickwell Bury, Biggleswade, Bedfordshire, SG18 9EF is a residential yoga centre offering courses of varying length and intensity. Tel: 01767 627271.

Further Reading

Parts One & Two

Practical Ayurveda: Secrets for Physical, Sexual and Spiritual Health by Atreya, Weiser

The Handbook of Ayurveda by Dr Shantha Godagama with Liz Hodgkinson, Kyle Cathie

Ayurveda: The A–Z Guide to Healing Techniques from Ancient India by Nancy Bruning and Helen Thomas, Dell

Supplement Bible: Hundreds of New Natural Products that will help to Improve your Mind and Body Fitness by Earl Mindell, Ph.D, Thorsons

Perfect Healing: The Complete Mind/Body Guide by Deepak Chopra, MD, Bantam

A Life of Balance: The Complete Guide to Ayurvedic Nutrition and Body Types with Recipes by Maya Tiwari, Healing Arts Press

Ayurveda: The Ancient Indian Healing Art by Scott Gerson, MD, Element

Ayurveda for Women: A Guide to Vitality and Health by Dr Robert E. Svoboda, David & Charles

Absolute Beauty: Radiant Skin and Inner Harmony through the Ancient Secrets of Ayurveda by Pratima Raichur with Marian Cohn, HarperCollins

The Complete Book of Ayurvedic Home Remedies by Vasant Lad, Piatkus

Part Three

A Simple Celebration: A Vegetarian Cookbook for Body Mind and Spirit by Ginna Bell Bragg and David Simon, Harmony Books

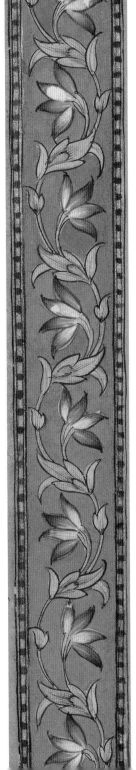

The Healing Energies of Water by Charlie Ryrie and David Cavagnaro, Gaia Books

The Ayurvedic Cookbook: A Personalized Guide to Good Nutrition and Health by Amanda Morningstar with Urmila Desai, Lotus Press

The Complete Book of Ayurvedic Home Remedies by Vasant Lad, Piatkus

The Handbook of Ayurveda by Dr Shantha Godagama, Kyle Cathie Ltd

The Healing Cuisine: India's Art of Ayurvedic Cooking, by Harish Johari. Healing Arts Press

Healing with Whole Foods: Oriental Traditions and Modern Nutrition by Paul Pitchford, North Atlantic Books

A Life in Balance: The Complete Guide to Ayurvedic Nutrition and Body Types with Recipes by Maya Tiwari, Healing Arts Press

Indian Food: A Historical Companion by K. T. Achaya, Oxford University Press

Further information is available from:

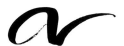

Bharti Vyas Holistic Therapy and Beauty Centre
5 & 254 Chiltern Street
London W1M 1PF

www.bharti-vyas.co.uk
(helpline) 020 7486 7910
Fax: 020 7224 3382

Index

acne 47, 59, 62, 73, 74

ageing 55

Air 8, 12, 27–30

  body tissues 58

  foods to balance 170–2

  health problems 24–5, 30

  menopausal symptoms 66

  menstrual cycles 61

  questionnaire results 22–3

  skin care programme 48–55

  specific natural elements
    68–70

  stress 56–9

  yoga exercises 28, 89

almonds 52, 65, 74, 81, 105,
  168

aloe vera 34, 61–3, 66, 68,
  75–6, 79, 83

amber 72

amla 130

angelica 83

anxiety 11, 69, 75

aphrodisiacs 127–32

apples 76, 78

apple crystal 167

aromatherapy 106

arthritis 69, 72

asanas see yoga

ashwagandha 69–70, 123, 130

athlete's foot 75

avocado 54

Ayurveda

  creation myth 13

  introduction 4–16

  origins 12

Ayurvedic

  clinics 181

  ingredients 179

  meditation and yoga 182

  organizations 182

  retreat 180

  supplements 68–73, 179

  tonics 123

baking soda 75, 78, 79, 80, 82

bananas 54, 76, 77, 78

basil 72

bay leaf 80

beauty 11, 46–55

bergamot 53

besan flour 55

beverages 153–4

bhringaraj 71

blackheads 75

blood letting 10

body

  purification 104–23

  tissues 58, 69

boswellin 72

bowel problems 11

breasts, sore 63–4

breath, bad 75

breathing 82, 84

buckwheat recipes 147, 160

calcium 61, 65

camomile 83

camphor 53, 77

canola oil 51, 54, 105

cardamom 34, 65, 75, 78, 80,

carrots 65

castor oil 76, 105

cedar wood 72

cellulite 76

chakras 86–8

Charaka Samhita 7

cheese 65, 145, 162, 166

cherries 61–2, 78, 81

chest pain 77

chocolate 79

cholesterol 73, 80

cinnamon 65, 68

circulation, poor 81

cleansing and purification 6, 114–23

clove 53

coconut 34, 58, 65, 78, 79, 105

cod-liver oil 81

coffee 48

cold sores 76

colds and flu 76

comfrey 83

common ailments 74–83

conception 133

constipation 59, 61, 76

coriander 53, 74, 76, 77, 79, 81

corn oil 51, 54, 82, 105

coughing 77

couscous with goat's cheese 162

crêpes

  mushrooms *en crêpe* 163

  savoury 148

cumin 53, 62–3, 74, 77, 79, 81

curry leaves 77, 81

cystitis 77

dahl 152

dandruff 77

dashamoola tea 61, 121

date and almond slices 168

depression 69

dermatitis 48

detoxification 105–24

dhatus see body tissues

diabetes 59, 77

diarrhoea 77

diet 11, 66–7

disease, causes 15

dizziness 78

dosha 8, 12–13, 68

  balancing kit 105–6

  doshic mix 14

  questionnaire 17–26

Earth 8, 12, 38–43

  body tissues 58

  foods to balance 176–8

  health problems 24–5

  menstrual cycles 61–2

  questionnaire results 22–3

  skin care programme 48–55

  specific natural elements 72

  stress 56–9

  yoga exercises 42, 89

eczema 48, 59, 73

emotional distress 6

enema 120–1

energy elements 11–12

epilepsy 59

Epsom salts 76

essential oils 28, 34, 53, 54

eucalyptus 53, 71, 80

exercise 22–3, 65

eyes, puffy 58, 81

face

  massage 112

  softening mask 55

  see also skin

fasting 15

fatigue, chronic 11

feet, sore 81

fennel 34, 74, 75

fever 78

figs with paneer cheese 166

Fire 8, 12, 32–6

  body tissues 58

  foods to balance 173–5

  health problems 24–5

  menstrual cycles 61–2

  questionnaire results 22–3

  skin care programme 48–55

  specific natural elements 71

  stress 56–9

  yoga exercises 34, 89

fruit beverages 153

garlic 68, 77, 83

gas and flatulence 78

geranium 28, 53

ghee 53, 62, 75, 76, 78, 143

ginger 53, 62, 65, 68, 75, 76, 78, 80, 82

gingseng 72

(Indian) *see* ashwagandha

ginkgo biloba 71

goat's cheese, couscous and
    roasted vegetables 162
gotu kola 71
gout 72
guarana 72
guggulu 63, 132

hair lustre oil 58
hangover 79
haritaki 132
headaches 79
healing, body, mind and soul
    45–135
health problems 11, 12, 24–5
heart disease 59
heartburn 80
heavenly compress 121–2
herbal
    packs 11
    powder, cleansing recipes 52
honey 77, 82
hormones 49, 56
HRT treatments 64
hypertension 59

immune dysfunction 11
indigestion 80
inflammatory diseases 59
insomnia 11, 61, 69–70, 80

jasmine 28

kama dudha 66
kapha see Earth

karella 77
kidney problems 59
kumari 63, 132
kutki 62

lavender 53
lemons 52–4, 56, 72, 79
lentil
    dahl 152
    patties with roasted
        vegetables 164
lettuce 83
lime juice 67, 77, 78, 80, 82
liquorice 34, 68
liver disease 59

mangista 73
mango juice 75
marama 11
massage 11, 63, 105–23
massala spice powder 58
medical theory 69
meditation 28, 34, 42,
99–103
menopause 64–7
menstrual cycles 61–4
menstruation, period pains
    81
mineral supplements 67
mint 53
mushrooms en crêpe 163
musta 62, 64
mustard 78, 81, 105
myrrh 68

nasal scenting 121
neem 51, 73, 77
neroli 53
nutmeg 63, 75, 78, 81
nutrition 136–42

ojas (body tissue) 69
oleation 123
olive oil 105
oranges 52, 75, 79
osteoporosis 61, 64, 65–6

panchakarma see cleansing
paneer cheese 145
    figs with 166
papaya 54, 80
parsley 76
patchouli 53
peaches 76
pepper, black 62, 77
peppermint 71
period pains see menstruation
physical deterioration 6
pineapple 54, 76
pippali 62
pitta see Fire
pizzas, mini buckwheat 160
pomegranate juice 67
prakriti 8
prana 11
prawns, sweet and sour 165
primrose oil 81
prunes 76
psoriasis 48, 59, 81

punarnava 62, 64, 123
purging 120
purvakarma see detoxification

questionnaire 17–21

rasayana 6
recipes *see* subject headings
rejuvenation 6
rheumatism 81
rice 146
Rishis 5, 7, 47
rock salt 34
rosacea 59, 74
rose 56, 58, 68, 72
rosewater 56, 58

saffron 53, 65
St John's Wort 69
salad, beet and egg 161
sandalwood 34, 51, 53, 71, 75
sandwiches, roasted vegetable 159
scalp massage 110
scones 147
seasonal routines 25
sesame 28, 34, 51, 52, 54, 66, 77, 78, 81, 82, 105, 120
sexuality 124–33
shanka bhasma 66
shatavari 62–4, 66, 69, 123, 132
shirodhara see heavenly compress
sinuses 80, 81

skin
  blackheads 75
  care programme 50–5
  complaints 11
  dry 78
  face massage 112
  face softening mask 55
  fruit mask 54
  moisturising 54–5
  nourishing 52–3
  quick cleanser 57
soup
  bouillon 155
  carrot 158
  clear vegetable 156
  parsnip and courgette 157
soy
  beans 65
  milk 65
steam 11
stings, bee and wasp 75
strawberries 54
stress 56–9, 82–3
sunburn 83
sunflower oil 51, 54, 82, 105
supplements 68
sweat therapy 115–16
sweet potatoes, roasted 151

Tai Chi 22
tea 48, 81
tea tree oil 75
throat, sore 82
tomato salsa 144
tongue, furry 78

toothache 83
tridosha type 24
triphala 28, 73, 120
turmeric powder 55, 68, 73, 82

ubvartan scrub 106

vaginal dryness 66
vanilla 53, 68
vata see Air
Vedic texts 5
vegetables, roasted 149, 159, 162, 164
vetiver 34, 71
vidari 66
virchana see purging
vitamin E 81

walnut angels 169
water
  importance of 118, 139–41
  retention 62
wheat germ 105
winter cherry *see* ashwagandha
witch hazel 81
women, and Ayurveda 60–73

yam 66
yeast infections 62
ylang ylang 53, 71
yoga 11, 28, 34, 42, 66, 84–99
  breathing exercises 95–8
  postures 93–4
  sun salutation 90
yoghurt 55, 79